In Clinical Practice

For further volumes:
http://www.springer.com/series/13483

Taking a practical approach to clinical medicine, this series of smaller reference books is designed for the trainee physician, primary care physician, nurse practitioner and other general medical professionals to understand each topic covered. The coverage is comprehensive but concise and is designed to act as a primary reference tool for subjects across the field of medicine.

Şerefnur Öztürk

Neurological Disorders in Clinical Practice

Case Histories for Medical Students and Residents

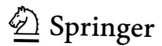 Springer

Şerefnur Öztürk
Faculty of Medicine
Department of Neurology
Selcuk University
Selcuklu
Konya
Turkey

Translated by Mehmet Ulu

ISSN 2199-6652   ISSN 2199-6660   (electronic)
In Clinical Practice
ISBN 978-3-319-23167-9   ISBN 978-3-319-23168-6   (eBook)
DOI 10.1007/978-3-319-23168-6

Library of Congress Control Number: 2015955258

Springer Cham Heidelberg New York Dordrecht London

Printed on acid-free paper

Springer International Publishing AG Switzerland is part of Springer
Science+Business Media (www.springer.com)

To my mother who has shaped me.

Foreword

This is a delightful book drawn from close observations of an experienced neurologist, looking at the effects of neurological diseases on daily lives. The presentation of the evolution of the conditions to readers is an art, which needs a great deal of compassion and depth of knowledge into the symptoms of neurological dysfunction.

To the general reader it gives the clear impression of the impact and consequences of early and late symptoms as well as ways of coping with and treating various conditions.

To medical students, it is a delight to read as it provides an excellent start on the long road ahead, on how to understand and empathize with their patients and their families.

To the medically qualified non-neurologists, there is a feel of what it is like to have a neurological condition and the effects of that on daily life. The reader will appreciate the subtleties and at times devastation inflicted by neurological diseases.

To the neurologists whether they are in training or in practice, it is an excellent reminder of what their patients experience in their daily lives. It is a great reminder to all to not put labels on individual patients. What these well-described narratives tell us is that not all those with say epilepsy or Parkinson's are the same, but they are totally different individuals who will need to be managed individually.

Professor Şerefnur Öztürk has captured all the presentations and dealt with management of major neurological conditions in a manner of a narrative relating to daily experiences, which gives all readers the chance to better understand the essence of neurology. For that she is congratulated.

Raad Shakir, MBChB, MSc, FRCP, FEAN
President of The World Federation of Neurology
London, UK
July 2015

Preface

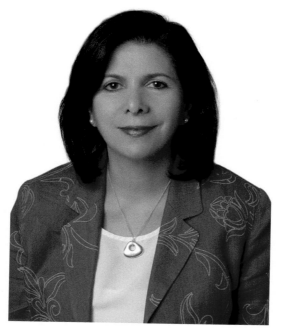

PROF. ŞEREFNUR ÖZTÜRK

The history that will be elicited from the patients and relatives of the patients is of great significance in the diagnosis of neurological diseases. Every doctor, every neurologist in particular, must be a good detective at the

ix

same time. The clues included in the histories of patients may often be more useful and guiding than sophisticated tests and examinations that will be conducted. The neurologist must also be a good listener. The patient needs to be investigated and evaluated within their entire social and physical environment. This is very important in both diagnosis and follow-up of treatment and at the same time will prevent the patient from being perceived as just a hospital file number. Understanding the individual's place and roles at work, in the home, in the family, and in the circle of friends will greatly influence the approach to the diagnosis of the disease and the process of examination, treatment, and follow-up. It must always be remembered that the patient is a spouse, a mother, a son, or a friend. These emotions are expressed in images designed by an artist.

In this book, while I was writing about the neurological processes which patients experienced and which are commonly observed in neurological practices, I made a special effort to present the personal characteristics, as well as home, workplace, family, and social circle characteristics in the histories of each patient by creating small-scale real-life stories. I intended to have each patient evaluated as a beloved mother, an admired friend, or a young person with ideals and thus create feelings of empathy towards him or her. In this way, I tried to ensure learning of neurological symptoms and findings, which appear affecting the lives of individuals in real life, in a more permanent and systematic manner. These stories bear traces from all of my patients and are a sum total of the impressions they have left on me. I made an effort to be able to convey what I have learned from my patients to my students and my colleagues.

I would like this book, which also bears a sentimental value for me, to serve as a useful tool in learning the symptoms of neurological diseases.

As Sir William Osler put it, "Listen to your patient; he is telling you the diagnosis."

Selcuklu, Konya, Turkey   Şerefnur Öztürk

Acknowledgment

I would like to thank my mentors who encouraged me to be a doctor and especially a neurologist, my parents and especially my grandmother who have supported me, my colleagues and friends who shared my ambition to make new projects, my patients who have trusted me and allowed me to touch their lives, my students who have motivated me by their learning passions, Assoc. Prof. Lale Avsar, who designed pictures to increase the artistic component of this book, Prof. Bulent Ozturk, who has supported me not just as my husband but also as a friend and a colleague, and my son Özgün Erinç, who has trained me to understand all stages of life.

Finally I would like to thank the Springer Team (especially Joanna Bolesworth) for their support during the publishing of this book.

Contents

Chapter 1
Parkinson's Disease

Altan opened his eyes when he heard the steps of his daughter who had just entered the room. Aysel knew that her father had been suffering from exhaustion in the daytime and sleeplessness at night. Therefore, she tried not to enter the room where her father was sleeping or even not to turn on the TV lest he woke up because she knew that he had difficulty getting into sleep. She had realized from the half-eaten slices, heated dishes, and other traces that her father had spent time in the kitchen at night. Her father, who used to be a very tidy and neat person, had begun to leave the kitchen unexpectedly messy recently. There were always bread crumbs around, and food remains scattered on the counter or on the table. She thought it best not to say anything to him again. Her father had grown sulky recently, or so she thought. He did not accept what was told him and got irritated immediately.

When Altan opened his eyes, Aysel winced as if she had been caught unawares and said, "Dad, sorry, I was washing the clothes and had to enter to get your laundry." Altan did not understand why his daughter had apologized but what he was sure of was that he was cheerless again. Yes, he had never been the same himself after his wife's death, but he had been feeling quite morose and lacking in energy during the past few months. "Well, I am no longer a young boy at age 68, ha?" he thought. They had been repeating this sentence at every meeting he had with his friends, yet still the others seemed to

Ş. Öztürk, *Neurological Disorders in Clinical Practice:*
Case Histories for Medical Students and Residents,
In Clinical Practice, DOI 10.1007/978-3-319-23168-6_1,
© Springer International Publishing Switzerland 2016

be better and healthier than him. At least, all of them were very eager to attend those meetings. For Altan, on the other hand, those meetings were like a burden. His friends, who had noticed the situation from his manners, had assigned this task to Aysel. No matter what, she would convinced Altan and take him to his friends. This was also good for Aysel because she felt more free, thinking that her father was having a good time, too.

"Ouch, my shoulders!" he whined. "Oh, God, it seems as if I am carrying the whole world on my shoulders. It is in vain whatever I do about it." Aysel responded from the corner, "If you like, I will put a hot towel on them!" "No dear," Altan replied. "I tried many things last week but alas they did not work. These pains will almost confine me to bed. It has become like a ceremony for me to rise from the bed. You see, it looks as if they will have to scrape me off the bed." His mind had drifted past once again; he used to be so nimble that when he moved, those around him seemed to be trying to take care of themselves.

Aysel looked with compassion at her father, who appeared to be daydreaming. "Come on, dad. It is all because you are tiring yourself out. I will not allow you to go to the garden again," she said. "Alright, alright, like mother, like daughter," he smiled.

Indeed, even getting up had become difficult for him. His entire body moved like a metal nugget. It felt as though his whole body had been frozen or covered with something hard. Fortunately, things were getting better after he moved for a while. He made for the bathroom with slow steps, his painful shoulders still in his mind. When he was through with the toilet, he walked to the sink to wash his face and hands. The face he saw in the mirror seemed not to belong to him. "How tired I look," he said to himself. He reached for the soap, but the first washing with the soap did not make him feel clean enough. His skin felt slimier now. He moved the soap in his hands once again until it had produced adequate foam then rubbed the foam all over his face elaborately and rinsed finally. Now, he felt better. He combed his hair and went to get dressed, without shaving. Shaving had also begun to prove difficult for him recently. No matter how much care he took, he could not adjust the razor properly and left the bathroom as if he had just returned from a fight. The cotton pieces he put on the cuts on his face elated Aysel and she teased him saying, "Oh, dad, you look like a snowman again." He thought, "This is a good girl, look how well she teases me without hurting!"

The breakfast table would be laid before he came. Since Aysel, too, had to go to work early, she woke up earlier her father and laid the table. Though hurriedly prepared, than table always had foods that contained the basic nutrition. Especially, eggs were invariably ready at the table. This was a habit Aysel had inherited from her mother. She used to say, "One must eat an egg every morning!"

Altan first took a sip from the tea before him. "Thank you!" he said to her, "It has made me feel good!" and at the same time watched his daughter put some bread, cheese, and egg on her plate. He did not feel like eating anything, but if he refused to eat, Aysel would again make a face. So, he took a slice of bread, turned it over, and placed on the plate again. He picked up the egg and began to peel it, but it felt like a torture. After a while, he was unable to hold the egg properly and peel it. "Dad, you have so got used to laziness!" Aysel called to him, reaching for the egg in the meantime. She wanted to finish the job immediately and leave. "Here you are; your egg is ready!" she said, while leaving the egg on his plate. At the same time, she looked at her father's face, but there was no expression of joy or fury on it; indeed it seemed as though there was no expression on it. "Come on, dad! If only you expressed your feelings even if for once!" she thought. Altan did not use to demonstrate his feelings and emotional reactions either, but recently, it had seemed that he was making more of an effort to hide his feelings. It was hard to be able to read his feelings from his face. Once, he had not laughed at a joke made by his friends and they had teased him, saying, "With this face of yours, you would make a good poker player, Altan." This change was not unknown to him either. It was as if the person who looked at him in the mirror was not himself but his same self with a mask on his face.

"I am leaving dad," called Aysel. "Good-bye," he replied, raising his hand from under the table and waving it. His hands, especially the right one began to shake if it remained motion-less for a long time. This shaking was not very severe but disap-peared when he moved it, but still he did not like people seeing his hand shaking. So far, he had managed to hide this situation even from Aysel. When shaking began, he hid his hand some-where or put it in his pocket on the other side or placed it under a cover. He could behave more freely now that his daughter had gone. He picked up the fork which had been lying before him for some time and directed it towards the slice of cheese. He had finally managed it, though with some difficulty. He finished his breakfast, picked up his newspaper from the corner where it had been thrown, and browsed through the pages. He did want to stay inside today; he was feeling some-what depressed. Why don't I go to the garden? He thought. He wanted to go to the toilet before he went out, but it was impos-sible. This constipation will kill me, he thought. It seemed as if it was getting worse. He put on a cardigan, and before he set out for the garden a few blocks away, he scribbled a message for his daughter on the notepad on the table, saying he was going to the garden and would be back in the evening. He shut the door behind him and left. He walked as he watched around. It appeared to him that everything around had accelerated. He felt like he was in a fast-forward film. Oh, what is this haste? What are they trying to catch? He thought. By this time, he had arrived at the garden. He noticed that the gate to it had not been closed completely, so he pushed it open. This garden, which he used jointly with his neighbor, was his little escapade. He relaxed there, away from all watching eyes, and passed time taking care of his flowers and a few fruit trees. He was over-joyed when he saw that the roses he had planted in the middle had blossomed. They looked so beautiful in yellows and pinks. He went near them to take in their nice smell, but they did not give off much smell. Today's roses are only for their appear-ance, he thought. What is the use of having roses without smell?

There were lavenders in the corner. Look, how beautiful they will smell, he thought. He bent down, broke off a few branches, and brought them nearer to his nose, but alas, they did not smell either. He left the barely smelling lavender branches on the ground. He had already grown tired. Fortunately, there were a few stools in the corners. He sat down and began to think. Everything was so different. When had all these differences begun? It was a few years ago when he first noticed the slight twitches in his hand. He had not paid much attention to it, thinking that it was because of tiredness, but whenever he started to relax in full, his hand began to remind itself. He had realized that when he held something in his hand, the shaking decreased. It was a piece of knowledge that benefited him. Whenever he realized that someone might understand the situation, he resorted to this trick and got over the problem. But what about the other changes? He had become as slow as a snail. He was feeling extremely tired for no apparent reason and his shoulders and back were aching. His appetite had disappeared. Did I really grow too old? He thought. But my friends are the same age as me. They are better than me. If only Sevim were alive, then I would not be like this. He was about to cry. While he was wiping his eyes, he realized when he tried to remove the saliva that had accumulated on the edge of his mouth that he had difficulty swallowing his saliva.

When Aysel came home, she called her father. When she got no response, she looked around and saw the note on the table. After she picked up the note paper, she noticed that it was a piece of clumsy writing informing her that her father was in the garden. As far as she knew, her father's handwriting was very beautiful. When had it become so? All of a sudden, she realized that this was not the only difference in her father. The shaking she noticed in his hand, slowing of his movements, lack of appetite, pains… "Could those be symptoms of a disease?" she thought. To her sorrow, she noticed that she had not thought over the problem due to the load of heavy work. They had dealt with the problems through temporary solutions but now perhaps something had to be done, she thought.

Yes, she would immediately go to hospital and get an appointment. Since there was shaking, it would be best to go to the neurology department. If it is not the right department, they will guide me, she thought. When she informed her father that they would go to hospital, as she had expected, he objected. "I have nothing to worry about, I am a little tired, that's all," he insisted. When he realized that his daughter would not give up, he had to consent.

Altan movements seemed to have become worse while they were going to hospital. Aysel noticed on the way that he had faltered for no apparent reason. It was as if he was frozen for a moment and then he was able to lift his foot off the ground with extreme difficulty and proceed. When they met the doctor, Aysel was as excited as Altan. While the doctor was asking his questions, Aysel noticed that he had indeed experienced all those things being described. When the examination finished, the doctor looked at both and said, "Altan, as a result of your descriptions and my examination, I think you suffer from Parkinson's disease. But in order to eliminate other possibilities, you will have to have a few additional tests."

Aysel looked at her father; Altan was listening to the doctor with an expressionless face again. As they were heading for the door, Aysel said, "Don't worry, dad! We will fight together. Altan looked at his daughter's face with hope and replied, "Yes, honey, yes, we will fight on."

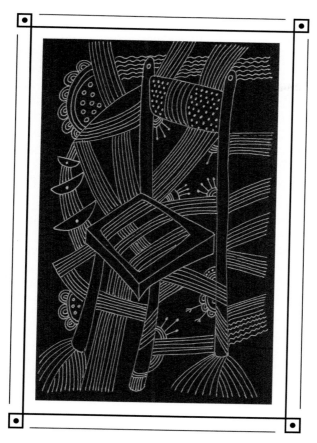

FIGURE 1.1 Inspirations and reflections from neurological phenomena (Image courtesy and copyright of Assoc. Prof. Lale Avşar, Selcuk University School of Art and Design, Turkey. Used with permission)

Chapter 2
Stroke

Like he had been doing since his retirement every day, Selim woke up early, first drank a large glass of water, and then, without even having his breakfast, left home to take his three-kilometer walk. His neighbors who saw him in the street had already begun to tease him saying, "Oh, Selim, you have started the day healthy again." Selim, on the other hand, continued his walk taking no heed of the jokes and replied, in his turn, saying, "The harmful effect of smoking for 40 years will disappear only in this way. I would advise you to do the same." Yes, the walking distance was really about three kilometers, but one kilometer of it was with normal walk and the remaining two kilometers were like torture. He had difficulty breathing and his heart was beating as if it was going to come out of his chest; he stopped and took a rest every 10 m, but he was persevering. He did not stop walking until he saw the shop with a yellow sign indicating the end of the 3 km course. It had been a year since he had retired and he needed a long life to do all the things he had postponed in his life. He had not done any exercise during the time when he worked and smoked a packet of cigarettes every day. He would eagerly await the fatty and sweet dishes his wife cooked as he did not feel full with the food served at the cafeteria of his workplace. His wife Meltem was a little plump but pretty lady who complained of her weight. She used to say, "Selim, we are getting old; we'd better eat lighter food. Look, I watch people on TV every day

Ş. Öztürk, *Neurological Disorders in Clinical Practice:*
Case Histories for Medical Students and Residents,
In Clinical Practice, DOI 10.1007/978-3-319-23168-6_2,
© Springer International Publishing Switzerland 2016

saying we should eat salads, vegetables, and fruit. They say they are better than medicine for all kinds of illnesses." However, Selim would reply, with some resentment, "Come on, Meltem, after all, I cannot eat a decent meal throughout the day; please, do not interfere in my food." Selim would become sluggish after every meal and have a headache. Meltem failed to discourage Selim from consuming excessive salt no matter what she did in this regard. Although she put very little salt in the dishes to reduce her own intake of excessive salt, the salt cellar kept its place handy on the dinner table as if it were his best friend. When she said, "Can your headache be due to salt? Look, our neighbor also complained of the same kind of headache, and when he went for a checkup, they diagnosed him with hypertension and they removed the salt stand from the dinner table," Selim would look at her resentfully, saying "Look, my dear, if you are comparing me to a man of 90 years old, then I have nothing to say to you."

Having finished his walk, Selim wanted to have a rest at the cafe on the corner. This time, he felt weaker and his head had already begun to ache. After he bought some sandwiches and biscuits for the household, he hailed the taxi on the corner. When he arrived home, Meltem met him with some worry in her face, "Why are you late, Selim? Did anything happen? You look much more tired today."

Selim went to the kitchen saying, "There is nothing wrong with me, I am fine." He was very hungry. He laid the table, adding the sandwiches, biscuits, and cheese to the side of the tea that had been already made. He felt palpitations in his heart throughout the breakfast. It was as if a bird was fluttering in his chest. "It is because I walked very fast," he thought, and he made an effort so that Meltem would not feel anything. He could not help thinking, "If she notices something, she won't allow me out."

After breakfast, he picked up his newspaper and went to his armchair. Suddenly, he staggered where he was, and while he was trying to hold the table, he caused the plate on it to fall to the ground. Meltem rose to her feet in panic and rushed to him. She held him by the arm, asking worriedly, "What happened, Selim? Are you alright?" and made him sit in the armchair. Selim said, "There is nothing, I am fine," but his words were barely audible. He had collapsed on the right side of the armchair. He noticed that he had difficulty raising his arm. Meltem was examining Selim's face with apprehension and at the same time trying to make him drink water from a glass she had filled. It was as though his mouth had become askew. She also had a lot of difficulty making him drink the water. "Let's wait for a while. If it still persists, then we need to see a doctor," she said in a hurry. Half an hour later, Selim felt better. He had managed to raise his arm and his speech too had become more understandable. "Oh, Selim, you really frightened me," said Meltem. "Anyway, it is gone now. Today, rest well; there will be no more walk whatsoever."

They had a quiet and uneventful afternoon. As she rose to cook the dinner, Meltem turned to Selim and said, "If you feel better, why don't you water the flowers in the balcony? That way, you will also get some fresh air."

Selim rose to his feet, filled a bucket with water, and walked to the balcony. Hardly had a minute passed when a thud was heard from the balcony. Having rushed to the balcony, Meltem found Selim on the floor, trying to rise up in the water spilt out of the bucket. His right side was immobile. He was making incoherent sounds and could not rise to his feet. It was as if Selim saw Meltem's anxious face but could not recognize her. His right arm was trying to move his leg but failed to do so. He wanted to say, "Let's see a doctor immediately," but words were coming out of his mouth which he himself could not understand. It was as though his right side did not exist at all and he did not feel anything. He had a terrible headache and he did not remember where he was and what he was doing. He seemed to have got lost in time and space. Everything grew dimmer a while later and his vision got worse; he felt as if his vision had been blocked by black barriers. Meltem tried to hold Selim's right arm and leg, which were moving about uncontrollably and noticed that the asymmetry in his face was becoming more distinct. At the same time, she was shouting to the next door neighbor for help. At last, the neighbor heard her and called in a hurry, "What happened Meltem? Where is Selim?" She replied, "Would you send for an ambulance, please? Selim is very bad."

An ambulance arrived half an hour later. When they were trying to place him on the stretcher, Selim's arm dangled lifelessly. Meltem could not help crying, saying, by the way, in sobs, "It is all because of me. If only I had not wanted him to water the flowers."

Tears had formed in Selim's eyes. It was as if he felt that he was at the beginning of a long and arduous path. The ambulance set off, with Meltem on board, too.

The ambulance first headed for the emergency service of the nearest hospital. When they arrived at the emergency service, the doctor there received the necessary information from Meltem and examined him quickly. Then he said, "He may have an embolism. He needs to be taken to a better equipped hospital." Selim was put in the ambulance once again and it set off again. Their destination this time was the emergency service of a university hospital. The patient was examined immediately. When they took Selim to the imaging unit, Meltem began to better understand the gravity of Selim's situation. She started to wait quietly. For a moment, she wanted to take out her phone and call their daughter, who lived in another city. But, what could she say right now? So, she gave up the call. Time lingered on. Meltem was trying to figure out where they had made a mistake and thought over every minute of their past few days. At last, Selim appeared at the door. The technician next to him looked sorry. Meanwhile, the doctor who examined the films on the screen approached Meltem. The doctor, who she deduced to be a neurologist, talked hurriedly to the emergency unit doctors. Two hours had passed in the meantime. It seemed as if Selim's situation was deteriorating. The neurologist asked her about when and how the incident took place as well as his habits and history of illnesses. He was surprised by the fact that the family had no prior information of Selim's having hypertension. When he said, "His blood pressure is very high at the moment. It probably rose occasionally in the past. If only you had had it measured now and then," Meltem shook her head in grief, "Oh, doctor, I told him to do so many times, but he never took heed of me." "Okay, easy, easy, do not be sad," the doctor said. "The damage is done. Now we will do our best. Fortunately that you arrived fast without delay. It is only three and a half hours since the incident took place. The patient may have a chance for recovery, so we must act immediately." Then, he turned to Meltem and said, "We think that your husband has embolism in his brain. In other words, he is having a stroke at the moment. We will have his brain imaging and blood tests soon, and if we deem it appropriate, we will give him an effective drug, which is thrombolytic therapy. This treatment will significantly increase your husband's chance of recovery. Has he had a stroke or a serious accident that affected his head in the past three months? Has he had a tumor, a serious operation in the head, or an important brain disease? Have doctors ever talked about an anomaly in his arteries before? Which medicine has he been on? Has he been using a medicine like warfarin, aspirin, and the like?" Mrs. Meltem tried to answer the questions on the one hand and looked at Selim, who was gradually becoming more and more sleepy. "Please, do whatever you will do immediately; he is getting worse on the other. Please hurry up." Meanwhile, the doctor was ordering around and said that he wanted to see the results of the laboratory tests as soon as possible and that a thrombolytic drug should be prepared.

He approached Meltem with a paper in his hand and began to tell her about the situation.

"An embolism has occurred in your husband's brain. There is no blood flow in a sizeable area in the brain. Fortunately enough, however, you were able to come on time and this enables us to give thrombolytic treatment. As far as we gather from the responses to the questions we asked you, there is no obstacle before us to perform this treatment. However, you need to give your consent."

Meltem was now in greater panic. "How come? Why do you need to get my consent? Is this a harmful treatment?" The doctor explained calmly: "This is the most effective treatment that can be used to cure our patient, and it is a proven one. However, some side effects may arise. And the most importantly there may be bleeding. But we will do our best to prevent this from happening."

Mrs. Meltem had now better understood the situation. "If only I had my daughter with me now," she thought, but there was nothing to do. She read the form given to her and said, "Yes, I consent. Please, start as soon as possible."

The patient was immediately taken to the intensive care unit in the neurology department. Everything had already been made ready. They began the treatment instantly. Everything seemed on the monitors. Mrs. Meltem was waiting quietly outside the intensive care ward. The intensive care doctor came out an hour later and said that the treatment had been completed, that they had to keep the patient under constant control, and that he had to spend the night in the neurology intensive care ward, adding they could see the patient an hour later.

An hour later, Mrs. Meltem was in the intensive care ward at the bedside of the patient. She thought that the place was extremely disorderly. There were screens, cables, and things she had never seen before everywhere.

She whispered softly, "Selim." Selim opened his eyes as if he was waking up from sleep and stared at Meltem for some time. "How are you, dear?" asked Meltem. Selim raised his hand slightly from the bed and began to squeeze Meltem's hand as though he would never let go of it. Two drops of tear began to fall down from Meltem's eyes, while the nurses looked at them, thinking what that lovely couple might have experienced.

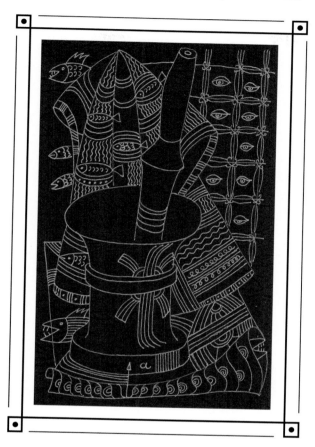

FIGURE 2.1 Inspirations and reflections from neurological phenomena (Image courtesy and copyright of Assoc. Prof. Lale Avşar, Selcuk University School of Art and Design, Turkey. Used with permission)

Chapter 3
Multiple Sclerosis

Pelin was squinting at the book in her hand, all attention but still failed to focus fully on the image. Then, she remembered to look at the page with a single eye at a time. First, she covered her right eye with her hand and noticed that the page she looked at with her left eye was quite clear and the writings were fairly legible. Then, she covered her left eye and tried and noticed that it was as if there was a frosted glass before her eye. She rubbed her eye thoroughly but it was of no avail. She tried to look again, but colors were also indistinguishable and she felt as if she were in a pale and misty world. As she moved her eye, she felt a pain somewhere deep inside, too. She had experienced such a thing two years ago for the first time. She never forgot it; when she woke up in the morning, she could not see the room clearly. She went to the bathroom, thinking that it would straighten out when she washed her face, but she could not see her face clearly in the mirror. Washing her face had not worked, either. All the same, she did not mind and thought that it would disappear soon. The situation had not changed for two days, but she had spent those two days trying not to make anyone feel it. Her colleagues had realized that there was something strange, but Pelin had managed to evade their questions, saying she had a headache, leaving early and postponing her duties. Indeed, the problem with her vision had disappeared gradually within two days.

Ş. Öztürk, *Neurological Disorders in Clinical Practice: Case Histories for Medical Students and Residents*, In Clinical Practice, DOI 10.1007/978-3-319-23168-6_3, © Springer International Publishing Switzerland 2016

Pelin was a very disciplined, hardworking, and popular person at her workplace. She had a large group of friends, too. She was a cheerful, active, and compatible friend. They would often organize trips and visit different cities together. Generally, she did not worry about her health, and she did not even remember when she had last seen her doctor. Of course, she had occasional problems, but she did not take them seriously, thinking that anyone might have such problems and considered them natural. Indeed, her health problems would not last long and finished in the end. She had suffered a vertigo-like thing a few times, and she had felt as if she were walking on cotton. Her friends who saw her walking falteringly had teased her, saying that she was walking like an intoxicated person but although she had not taken alcohol, her situation continued for a few days. She took a few days off, attributing her condition to fatigue and rested at home. She never forgot that once, too, she had seen two lampposts although there was one only; she had kept blinking her eyes, but the lampposts remained two. When she told her friends of her condition, they did not take it seriously either and they teased her, saying come on, you are lucky, you have twice as many friends as you had now. Her seeing double, which occurred especially when she looked left, got right when she looked at the center. Everything had straightened again within three or four days. However, the vision was more indistinct today and this caused Pelin to be worried slightly. Unfortunately, it was a holiday. First, she wanted to call her mother. When she picked up her phone, she could not see the keys well, but fortunately she had recorded the number in speed dialing. When her mother answered, she made an effort not to worry her, saying "Mum I had a headache. I thought it would disappear soon but it did not. Would you please come to me?" Her mother knew that Pelin would not exaggerate trivial matters. She asked with some apprehension if there was something serious. She remembered that Pelin had also complained of numbness in her right side a few months ago. She had not mentioned this either; only she had been surprised when she was able to hold the plate that had just been taken out of the oven without hesitation and without feeling hurt. When her mother had asked, "Don't you feel pain in your hand Pelin?" she had responded "no," but when she had touched the plate with her other hand, she had pulled her hand back in pain, thus noticing the loss of feeling in her right side. Fortunately, this situation had also vanished in a week, and Pelin had not gone to see a doctor despite all her mother's insistence. But, what had happened during that week had always remained in her mother's mind. She always remembered a woman she had met at a meeting with friends. She was a beautiful woman of 40 but whenever she rose to her feet, she staggered and had difficulty drinking her tea due to a visible shake in her hands. She had wondered how a young person had that condition. She had met a few people with Parkinson's disease, but they were old people. She had wondered if it was in the family but had not dared to ask. What kind of a disease was that? The young woman often forgot her landlady's name, and while she talked, she confused the order of events. As far as she had gathered, she had been suffering from that condition for years, and when she frequently got up to go to the toilet, the other guests sighed with sorrow. She had not stayed long there; she had got up to go home, but whenever she remembered that woman, she realized what a blessing it was even to be able to walk properly.

Pelin, too, was experiencing various problems; she knew that, but for her, no disease would suit her daughter. On their last holiday, Pelin had entered the bathroom, saying "Mum, I will take a hot bath!" but when she had come out, she had slowed down and looked at her with a squint in her eyes. She had picked up her book but put it back immediately. It was obvious that something was going wrong, yet Pelin just said she was feeling sleepy and went in and slept. Fortunately, she was more cheerful when she woke up and there seemed to be no problem. However, various problems, though they were temporary, that crossed her mind alarmed Pelin's mother. Without asking further questions, she said she was coming. When she arrived at Pelin's house, she immediately noticed that Pelin was sad and agitated. "What happened darling?"

she asked curiously. In the meantime, she was examining Pelin. Her motherly intuitions told her that there was something serious this time. Pelin hugged her mother and said, "Mum, don't worry; it is not something serious; I am just experiencing some problems with my sight. It will pass, but somehow I was frightened." Pelin also noticed something serious in her voice. It sounded hoarse and deep. When she examined her more closely, she saw that her left shoulder was lower and the movements in the left side of her face were fewer. "I am sure you haven't eaten anything. Let me prepare something." She said and headed for the kitchen. Pelin was feeling really weak. From where she was sitting, she called to her mother, "I won't eat much mum, don't bother!" Her mother came out of the kitchen with a tray in her hand. She had prepared a grand breakfast table again with a motherhood miracle. Pelin sat down willy-nilly. She began to cough at the first bite. She took a large sip from a glass, thinking that it would clear her throat, but it further increased her cough. It was as though the water was going to her lungs, not to her stomach. Agitated by this, her mother did not know what to do. In the meantime, Pelin, who had calmed down a bit, dreaded to take another sip but upon thinking of her mother's effort to prepare the food, she took another bite. The same thing happened; Pelin began to cough again like she was going to choke. This time, she was afraid to drink water, too. "Alright" said her mother, "we are going to see a doctor immediately. No objection. I haven't found my daughter in the street." Pelin tried to object, saying, "Come on mum, it will disappear." But she herself noticed the feebleness in her left arm. What was happening? Were all these things interrelated? Suddenly, she herself was in fear. While she was looking at her mother from where she was sitting, her memory drifted back to the past: loss of vision which she had experienced initially and subsequent problems she had suffered; blurred vision she had after every bath, which she was afraid to confess to herself; and other cases which she did not remember but caused her friends to nickname her "fragile princess"… Were all of them a part of a whole? If she could distinguish her mother's face, she would see that she was looking at her with tears in her eyes, but her concern was obvious even from her voice. "Alright, mum you are right. Let's go!" she said. When they got into the car her mother had called, she felt that a new era was beginning in her life. Her mother had thought that she could get help from a friend working at a public hospital. "Let's go to the emergency unit first. The rest, we will see," she said. When they arrived there, her mother had already talked to her friend, and a doctor in the emergency service had promised to help. When they found the doctor, Pelin was quite calm. They told the doctor what had happened. The doctor said, "We may not be able to do much in the present conditions of our emergency service; it may be an infection. Let's see your tests." When the test results came, the doctor told them, "As I have told you, the test results are normal. We may not find out much in the emergency, but since you have a problem with your eyes, I will refer you to an ophthalmologist." The mother had now been slightly relived. "Oh, thanks, it is not something urgent," she thought. They would go to an eye clinic first thing tomorrow. All of Pelin's complaints continued until the next day. Her mother did her best to make Pelin comfortable. She phoned her friends to tell them that she would not be able to come to work the next day.

When they got to the eye clinic, there were still a few hours before her examination. People of all ages were there waiting, those with covered eyes and those with thick glasses. When she entered the doctor's office, he asked what her problem was. "My vision has been blurred for three days," she said. "Do both your eyes have the same problem?" asked the doctor. "No, only the right one," she said. "But, I had had it in my other eye before." Her last words caused the doctor to divert his attention away from the monitor. "Did it happen before?" he asked again. Pelin thought to herself that it should be something important. "Yes," she said, "but it vanished within two to three days every time? "Did you have other complaints?" "How do you mean?" asked Pelin. "Like loss of strength, loss of balance, numbness," he replied. "Yes," Pelin said. "They occurred a few times but then all disappeared." The doctor examined Pelin's eye using a complex tool, measured her vision, and looked at her eye ground with a light-generating instrument. Finally, he said, "There is nothing wrong in the visible part of your eye." The mother felt relived at first but then asked, "Well, why does she have a visual impairment?" Pelin was looking at the doctor with as much curiosity. "I will refer you to a neurologist and they will do whatever is necessary," he said. Pelin hesitated, thinking, neurologist? Those who suffer from paralysis see a neurologist. Why should I go to the neurology department? Her mother's eyes had become wet again. The ophthalmologist tried to calm her down saying, "Don't worry, it may not be important but still needs to be investigated." Pelin and her mother headed for the neurology outpatient clinic. It was almost evening when they finally arrived at the neurology polyclinic. The neurologist had Pelin and her mother sit opposite him. Both looked very tired. He turned to Pelin and asked about her complaints to obtain information in addition to what he had learned from the consultation note. Pelin tried to tell him about her complaints, albeit feeling bored having to repeat the same things a third time. The doctor was listening with a serious expression in his face. She noticed that anything she said counted. All that staggering, visual problems, and seeing double seemed important. The doctor even asked if she had difficulty urinating. Indeed, yes, she herself had noticed recently that she had begun to go to the toilet very often. The doctor also asked some questions related to rheumatism. Did she have pains in her joints? Did she experience any problems concerning her skin and eyes? Pelin answered them one by one. Now and then, her mother interfered to make additions. During the examination, Pelin had become more aware of the weakness in her left arm, in addition to one in her eyes and her reflexes. When the doctor completed her examination, he said, "We need to keep you in hospital Pelin." Her mother got alarmed immediately. "Don't worry; these complaints of yours may appear in many diseases. We will have to have some tests done and especially we need to investigate your brain cerebrospinal fluid," said the doctor. "How do you mean?" asked

Pelin. "We will enter your spinal area in your back and take a small amount from the fluid flowing around the brain using a syringe. Then, we will send it to the laboratory for tests," he replied. Then, he added, "We will also have to examine your eye nerves. A detailed brain MR will be necessary, too. When all these are completed, we will have an idea about your illness." Pelin and her mother asked permission until the next day to get ready.

The following day, when they arrived at the hospital, they were ready for everything. The neurology service was a place where many kinds of patients stayed. Apparently, there were different patients and cases in each room. Some patients lay motionless. Some patients, on the other hand, were unexpectedly young. When Pelin moved to her room, she saw that there was another patient in the room. She was a young girl with a muscular disease who had come from a distant city. When Pelin had entered the room, she had stared at her, as if wondering why she had come. Then, she could bear it no longer and asked shyly, "Why did you come, sister?" Pelin did not want to reply. Instead, her mother responded, saying, "It is nothing my child, for tests only."

The next day passed with blood samples taken from the vein, brain MRs, and visual tests in laboratories. The day ended with taking of fluid from her back called lumbar puncture. In the meantime, the test results and her story were combined with the examination and a diagnosis began to shape up. The doctor explained to Pelin and her mother that their diagnosis of her condition was highly likely a disease called multiple sclerosis. He added, "But we will continue to explore other possibilities and we would like to start your treatment immediately. Don't worry! This disease does not progress in the same way in all patients. There is no reason for it to not progress better in your case." Pelin had begun to realize the situation now. Obviously, all those complaints of hers she had not paid attention to and the symptoms she was unable to explain were all symptoms of multiple sclerosis. Now, she knew and it was clear what she had to do next. She would be strong and not allow the disease to affect her life.

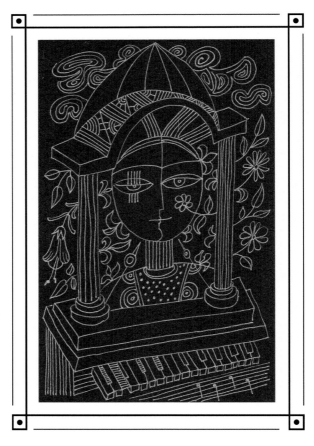

FIGURE 3.1 Inspirations and reflections from neurological phenomena (Image courtesy and copyright of Assoc. Prof. Lale Avşar, Selcuk University School of Art and Design, Turkey. Used with permission)

Chapter 4
Epilepsy

Sevgi finished high school. She decided to give the university exams another try and started to shuttle between the house and the test center. She lived a silent and routine life with her mother, father, and 5-year-old sister. She studied for school of law. Last year, she slightly missed her target. This year's preliminary assessment examinations were way better.

That morning, she woke up early as usual. They would take an overall assessment test at the test center. She quickly went through yesterday's notes. Meanwhile, her mother was trying to make something for breakfast. Come on my dear, eat something before you leave, she called her a second time. Seeing that her daughter did not care, she was both worried and angry. Sevgi was her precious one, who she first lost then gained back. Sevgi was three years old then. It first came with coughs, then the frothy drainage from the mouth and nose, and lastly that heavy fever. She couldn't get Sevgi's fever down, no matter what. Her body temperature remained over 39°. All of a sudden, Sevgi gazed at a point and her arms and legs started shaking. Her condition was getting worse as her mother shook her saying, "Sevgi my dear." She was stiffened. Her face started to get purple. She wasn't breathing. Her teeth were locked, and blood from the wound that she incurred on her lips while her mother tried to open her mouth mixed with her saliva, resulting in a frothy substance. "Sevgi my dear, please don't die,"

Ş. Öztürk, *Neurological Disorders in Clinical Practice: Case Histories for Medical Students and Residents*, In Clinical Practice, DOI 10.1007/978-3-319-23168-6_4, © Springer International Publishing Switzerland 2016

Melahat was struggling. She could do nothing; she couldn't manage to stop the convulsions. It was as if a century passed but Sevgi's convulsions weren't even abating. The next-door neighbor rushed in at Melahat's screams. When she got in through the semi-open door, she saw Sevgi go black and blue, with convulsions, and Melahat, who was struggling more than her. She immediately understood what was happening. Move away, Melahat, she is having a seizure, and she headed to the bathroom as she grabbed Sevgi. She turned on the big tap and she held the child under the water except for her head. She was simultaneously talking, "This is due to fever; we should make her cold immediately. My son Levent suffered many such seizures but fortunately, no damage is left." As she talked, the convulsions disappeared gradually, which was again longer than a century for Melahat, and Sevgi's face color was restored to normal. Melahat was very happy for regaining Sevgi as she looked at her sleeping pink-white face. From that day to this, Melahat was always scared to experience the same thing and started to care more for Sevgi, with an exaggerated attention. Sevgi knew this too; her mom told her to make sure she would be careful.

"Ahh mommy," she said in boredom. "I am already late, no time for breakfast. I'll have something to eat there; don't worry," she ignored.

Her bag was already prepared. She looked back at the ready breakfast table and her sad mom.

"Okay my dear, bye-bye," said her mom with a forced smile on her face.

Almost everyone were in their desks as she made it to the test center. She found an empty desk and sat down. A pencil, an eraser, and a handkerchief, yes everything seemed ready. "Water?" she looked around; there was no water in the bag and no candies, which were always there. "No matter," she said carelessly.

The question booklets were being handed out. She took her booklet. She immediately opened the first page and went through the page. The classroom started the test with the teacher's command, "You can start the test."

It was an easy one. She had to read question 20 once again. It was as if her mind was preoccupied with something and the question couldn't make it in. All of a sudden, everything was virtually lost. There was a crowd around her as she gained consciousness and they looked at her, worried. The teachers tried to get the students away but couldn't manage. Everyone was trying to understand what happened to Sevgi. Meanwhile, although she started thinking had that the exam was disrupted, and her efforts were wasted, the principal of the test center was trying to get that thought out of her mind and call the hospital. One of the teachers advised him to call ambulance. Meanwhile, Sevgi regained consciousness and look around with blank eyes. She could hardly grab the glass of water she was given, remembering nothing. She was only aware that all her body ached and she felt a heavy feeling of exhaustion. She could hardly have a sip from the glass of water that people around asked her to drink. It was sweet. The glass went empty after several sips. You eat nothing, and look what happens, the math teacher said reproachfully. Everyone felt comfortable when Sevgi sat down and said "Okay, I'm fine, I didn't have breakfast, this may be the cause," and everyone except the principal and several other teachers left the scene. "Okay, no need for an ambulance, the child is in a stable condition," said the principal to his secretary. "You can cancel the ambulance. It's better to inform her family," he called out.

Sevgi sat for a while and stood up, she then went into her classroom. Her friends acted as if nothing had happened. She started to pick up her books. She had a terrible headache and she was sleepy. Obviously she would feel much better if she went home.

She found a place to sit in the bus. She could make it home.

There was no one home when she arrived. Her mother had an arrangement with her friends. They had talked about it yesterday. She went straight to her room and lay on her bed.

It was almost dark outside when she woke up to her mother's voice. "Sevgi what happened my dear? what sleep is this," she said in worry. She sat up. She felt she was too hungry. "Nothing mom, the exam finished earlier, so I came home," she said. She anticipated what could happen if she told her she had passed out.

"Okay, get out of the bed and I'll get you something to eat," her mom said. The gloomy room hid her pale face from her mother. She made her way to the kitchen as she felt better.

The dishes looked delicious but their smell upset her stomach. With a sour face, she said, "there is a very bad smell, just like a burnt tire," looking at her face. "No, my dear, what tire? This is delicious stuffed grape leaves. You became way too picky," said her mom. She was in no mood to discuss. She closed her eyes and chewed several bites.

"Mom, I have too much homework to do," she said to her mother and headed to her room, but she could read just one or two pages before falling asleep again.

Melahat entered her room, saw her sleeping on her desk and touched Sevgi's forehead with worry. Oh, thank God, she had no fever whatsoever. They are pushing too hard on these children, she thought.

"Sevgi, my dear, come on, get into your bed now," she awoke her daughter. Putting on her pajamas as if she was in a dream, Sevgi could hardly make it to her bed.

She felt better as she woke up at the same hour in the morning. She quickly put on her clothes and washed her face; she had a slight pain but her mom noticed nothing yet. After yesterday's events, she couldn't escape from breakfast; she had some food to eat.

She felt okay on her way to the test center. That day, she had a heavy math class. In the second hour, the entire class was all ears, listening to the equations. All of a sudden, something strange happened on the blackboard. The numbers were twisting, growing, getting smaller, and moving. Sevgi opened her eyes wide. Sevgi's situation took the teacher's attention. "What's the problem Sevgi, anything you don't understand?" he asked. Sevgi did not reply him, so the teacher turned back to the blackboard. Then Sevgi started seeing normal numbers. She had a meaningless experience.

She thought this could be something from yesterday. Her stomach started to get upset. It was as if there was something moving upward from her stomach. Her color was paler. Luckily, it didn't last long. She didn't want to go out for the break time at the end of the class.

When she finally got back home in the evening, she again felt as nothing had happened. She planned to sleep later and catch up yesterday's unfinished topics. She looked at the test forms piled up on her desk. She had a coke and went to her desk. It was after three at night when she finally slept. She felt relaxed having finished her homework. When she woke up at the telephone's alarm in the morning, she was aware that she could not get enough sleep but she had to go to the test center. She got herself ready, made her breakfast, and left home.

At the fourth hour, she found it difficult to understand what the teacher was explaining. Again, things around were like moving, and the objects transforming their shapes. Suddenly everything disappeared again. Seeing Sevgi collapse on the desk, the teacher rushed in a hurry. The students next to Sevgi's desk also rose with worry. Sevgi was having convulsions, with her eyes fixed at a point. She was wheezing and she stated to go black and blue. She had foam in her mouth. Trying to move her, her friends noticed the wetness on the ground, which made them more worried. Sevgi kept having convulsions although many people around were trying to hold her. The teacher was helplessly holding her head to prevent her head from hitting the ground, but this did not have an end. Meanwhile, he was yelling around to make others call the hospital. Finally the convulsions disappeared and Sevgi's color began to restore to normal. He asked the secretary to call her family too. Sevgi was just laid on the desks. She opened her eyes but looked with meaningless eyes. She was again feeling pain in every part of her body, and she felt knackered. Her head was virtually empty. She tried to remember what had happened but to no avail. Some time later, she began to understand where she was and what was happening. She began crying when she heard her mother's voice. The teachers tried to relax the mother who rushed in asking what had happened. "It is all right, don't worry, she had a seizure, she is okay now," they said. Melahat suddenly staggered as she heard the word seizure. She was in panic. Her worst fears were confirmed; she remembered what the doctor told when she took Sevgi to the hospital when she was three. She struggled much to protect Sevgi but she doesn't listen to me, she thought.

She took her daughter immediately to the emergency unit of the hospital. The neurologist who was called to the emergency unit asked a number of questions to Melahat and Sevgi and finished her examination. Melahat was horrified by what she learned when the doctor said:

"Your daughter may have epilepsy but we have to make some tests; we can hospitalize your daughter." Sevgi and her mom hugged and looked at each other. "No more secrets between us Sevgi," said her mother hugging her. "Okay mom, no secrets!" she said, thinking about how she would cope with what she was to go through.

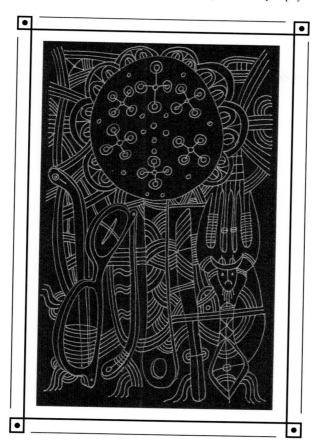

FIGURE 4.1 Inspirations and reflections from neurological phenomena (Image courtesy and copyright of Assoc. Prof. Lale Avşar, Selcuk University School of Art and Design, Turkey. Used with permission)

Chapter 5
Migraine

Bilge had woken up early, taken a hurried bath, got dressed, and had breakfast thinking that she would not last long without breakfast given her busy course schedule. She had examined the content of fridge quickly and laid the breakfast table with half-eaten cheddar cheese in a plate, some olives, a little jam, and two slices of bread. She would abstain from drinking tea and coffee on such busy days. She might experience that terrible pain again if she had too much tea and coffee. Bilge was a primary school teacher. She was teaching the third graders this year. She adored her job. Seeing the positive changes in her students' overall performance each year and even every day and witnessing their efforts to be become well-educated individuals made her happy. If only that annoying vice principal were not there. What a surly man he was. He made a mountain out of a molehill and drove everybody crazy. After every encounter with him, she had a terrible headache and her day would be ruined. As a matter of fact, she had the headache since her maidenhood. It occurred at least two or three times a month and lasted at least 2 or 3 days. When the pain came, she did not want to see anybody; any voice or sound was like a noise to her. She would keep the curtains of the classroom half closed as light also disturbed her extremely. Her little pupils who knew her situation would stop making noises immediately and try not to upset her. Initially, whenever their

Ş. Öztürk, *Neurological Disorders in Clinical Practice:*
Case Histories for Medical Students and Residents,
In Clinical Practice, DOI 10.1007/978-3-319-23168-6_5,
© Springer International Publishing Switzerland 2016

teacher's pains began, they felt guilty and therefore sorry. Then, their teacher explained the situation, saying it was not their fault but she would feel better if they kept quiet. On their part, they regarded those periods as periods of responsibility and tried to be as quiet as possible. Indeed, in an art class, one of her students had drawn the teacher with spiky hair, red eyes, and lightning in the sky. Bilge had been extremely moved when she saw the picture and thought that when these little individuals were properly taught, they understood things better than the adults. She still had difficulty describing her pain to her husband. She had discovered that her pain increased when she had old cheese, oranges, and fermented drinks like Berr and wine. Her husband insisted that she eat all kinds of cheese for breakfast and did not behave in an understanding manner when she wanted to retire to her room and sleep during the pain. But, a quiet room and sleep were the only things that best suited her during a fit of pain. When she woke up, she felt relieved. Although this situation affected the quality of her life to a great extent, she was trying to get by through such measures.

She ate breakfast quickly, drank her orange juice abundantly, and set off immediately. When she arrived at school, her students were already in. She heard a few students arguing in the corridor and went towards them, trying to understand what the problem was. The vice principal appeared in the distance. He approached with a sarcastic expression on his face and said "Mrs. Bilge, you are not able to control your students. You must exert more discipline on them". She began, "These are students from another class and I was only...," but the vice principal had already left there and slammed his door behind him.

Bilge was very proud of her class while she was making something for her class. When she entered the class, all the class was ready and greeted their teacher saying "Good morning."

The first hour went as usual. During the break, some of the students were in class and talking loudly. Bilge had not wanted to go to the teachers' room; instead, she had chosen to stay in class. She felt extremely tired. She had a slight nausea and it looked as if she did not know where she was. Slowly, that familiar pain began to give its first signs. Lines of light growing larger began to appear in front of her eyes. She had got used to those images which did not disappear even if she closed her eyes. She knew that those images would vanish 10–15 min later and her pain would set in. She sat on her chair without moving and with her eyes shut. Her students noticed the situation. Their teacher's face looked very pale. They all left the class to help her feel relieved. Bilge's pain began to spread to her left eye and the left side of her head. Sometimes, the pain began on the right side. It could also begin on both sides. This time, the pain was extremely intense. She started to feel sick. She tried to take control of herself but could not succeed. She vomited everything she had eaten. Her clothes and everything around her had become dirty. Another teacher who had heard the sounds entered the classroom. Seeing her in this state, he got worried. "Are you alright, Mrs. Bilge? What is wrong with you?" he asked in panic. Bilge was very embarrassed. She said "Nothing important, something that always happens. Only, this time I was more affected somehow." In the meantime, she was trying to wipe her face. "I will be OK if I get some rest," she said.

Orhan was surprised by Bilge's lack of concern. "How come? Won't you do anything about it? Don't you have medicine for it?"

"No, no," she shook her head. "Nothing important. It disappears when I sleep for a while and get some rest. Mum also suffered from the same pain. We are used to it."

Orhan could not understand. Why would not one go to see the doctor if they had such a problem? He remembered his wife; she would see the doctor at the slightest discomfort. Sometimes it was unnecessary, but in some cases, they had prevented certain diseases before they got worse. Therefore, he insisted, "We must see a doctor immediately; otherwise, it might do greater harm to you. Let's go and see what it is." They set out after they took permission from the vice principal. Upon learning Bilge's illness, the vice principal had expressed his concern and felt ashamed of his attitude in the morning. He said, "Don't worry; we will take care of your students. You go and finish your treatment."

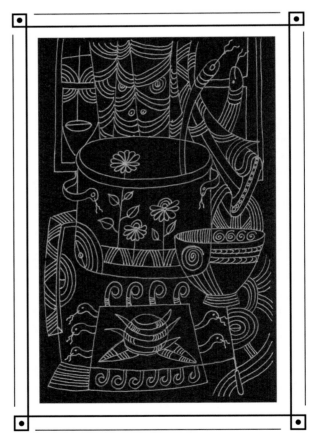

FIGURE 5.1 Inspirations and reflections from neurological phenomena (Image courtesy and copyright of Assoc. Prof. Lale Avşar, Selcuk University School of Art and Design, Turkey. Used with permission)

Chapter 6
Dementia

Sevil was looking at the television, which was playing away, with dreamy eyes on her usual couch. Meral, her daughter, switched the channel to her mom's favorite TV series. Once in a while, she would take her eyes away from her book to take a brief glance at the TV series, which had a rather slow pace. Moments later, she noticed that she was immersed into the book. She couldn't recall the female character's name although she knew the name well. "Mom, what was her name?" she addressed her mom. Sevil was suddenly startled from the image that preoccupied her mind. Her daughter repeated the question but Sevil kept looking in confusion. "Oh mommy, are you watching it or not?" Meral reproved. Sevil turned her face back to the television as if nothing happened. Minutes later, she stood up and began wandering the through rooms. Meral could hardly concentrate on the book. Her mom called her name from the next room. "Did you see my glasses my dear, I cannot find them." Meral felt obliged to stand up. "Mommy, you are already wearing them!" "My silly mind, just forgot them." Sevil went back to her couch. Meral tried to focus on her book but her mind was occupied with her mom's ever-increasing absent mindedness and forgetfulness. A few days ago, she forgot to take the keys, she was locked out, so she waited at the neighbor's house until and the evening, waiting for Meral to come. "Mom, why didn't you call me earlier"

Ş. Öztürk, *Neurological Disorders in Clinical Practice:*
Case Histories for Medical Students and Residents,
In Clinical Practice, DOI 10.1007/978-3-319-23168-6_6,
© Springer International Publishing Switzerland 2016

asked Meral but she couldn't give any answer. "All right mom, can you call my brother?" She had a set of spare keys. Her mom took the phone, and tried but somehow she couldn't manage to make a call. Oh, really, when was the last time her mom called her? It was way back. "Mom, what happened? Why aren't you calling me?" she asked. Her mom passed the phone with weariness. It was as if she was holding something she used for the first time. "Okay, I will call him," she said. When she took the phone back, she noticed that none of the dialed numbers were acquaintances and there were missing numbers. She called her brother and talked to him about the problem. Her brother lived in a distant neighborhood with his wife and two kids. "It'll take some time but I'll be there with my son," he replied.

Just as he said, he arrived in less than an hour. Showing up with his father, Efe jumped into his grandmother's lap as usual. Sevil was first surprised, and then she hugged her grandson too. Efe lost no time, "grandma, can you tell me about my grandfather's wartime stories?" he asked. Sevil seemed a little bit unwilling. Meral first upbraided her son, "Don't bother your grandma, don't you see, she is very weak," she said, but Efe was already pulling Sevil's arm. "Okay," said Meral, "but don't push her hard." Meanwhile, she reckoned that she could talk about the problem more comfortably with her brother. They went into the kitchen. Her brother, upset, looked curiously at Meral to understand why he was unexpectedly called away. He took her position reckoning that his sister would exaggerate the situation as she was always very much into details. "Yes," he said, "what made you worry so much?"

Meral's eyes immediately watered. "Mom has a dramatic change lately. She is no more the same; I suspect she hardly knows me at all sometimes. Don't you see, she doesn't take care of herself; she wouldn't even go out to throw the garbage away without fixing her hair. She keeps wearing the same dresses, and they are dirty, stained… This is not how my mom behaved. The house is messed up. Things are not in their usual places. The other day, I found my comb in the fridge; I thought I put it there by mistake but the glasses are in the bookshelf, shoes disorganized, drawers messy."

Her brother kept listening with some worry and more distress. Obviously, he didn't believe some of what she told him. "She is too old, what are you expecting her to be, to put on makeup and take to the streets? Of course, this is how it goes. You are exaggerating as always," he said, standing up. He needed a glass of water. He went to the cupboard, took a glass, but put it back; it was a dirty glass with deposits of grease. He gave it another shot but the result was the same. The shelf was full of dirty and clean glasses. He managed to find a clean one but his face suddenly blacked out. The entire neighborhood knew and rumored how meticulous his mom was. They suffered much as children because of her meticulousness. No one could enter the kitchen without washing their hands, and no glass was used twice. "But why?" he asked himself with grief. "So, she is not strong enough; we will have to find her a maidservant." Meral first looked at her brother with loving eyes. She said it's normal that he doesn't understand and accept the situation, she said to herself. He would never allow anyone to speak ill of her. And his mom was also very fond of him. She kept saying, my dear son, and would say nothing else. Meral was always envious of this mother-son alliance. "Well," he said, "maybe you are right. I will ask the neighbors to help us find a maidservant." His sister was smiling. Together, they went back into the living room. Efe was on his own, playing with something else. "So, the story is over," Meral asked Efe. "My grandma is skipping my favorite parts, so I quit," he replied. Sevil looked with startled eyes at the people in the room. She stood up, headed to her bedroom, and just lay on the bed. She was already asleep when Meral entered the room.

"Yes, my brother is right; maybe she is getting too tired,' she thought. As she put a blanket over her mother, she suddenly noticed that the roles had changed. It was always her mom who put blankets over them. She went straightaway to the next-door neighbor's house to arrange the maidservant.

The neighbor was a lady who was several years younger than her mom, suffering from many diseases but able to do the chores. She lived with her husband and unmarried daughter. She was pleased to see Meral and invited her in. Actually, she seemed as if she knew about it. "You are Meral, aren't you?" she asked. "I don't like her mood and how she behaves lately. We used to chat in the mornings but now she remains in the house; she hardly hears my hello. I thought she is upset with something, but there is nothing to be upset about. No one would knock on her door if it weren't for you. She smiles not and cries not; she just stands still."

Meral couldn't believe what she had heard. So, her mom was worse than she thought, but she should get this maidservant thing settled. "My mom is getting too tired; she is not strong enough to do the chores, and you know, we can only visit her once a week because of our work schedules. Could you arrange us a maidservant for my mom?" she asked.

"Sure," said Ayşe, "I'll arrange one immediately. I hope she is as you described and has no other problems." "Like what?" asked Meral, with surprised eyes. Ayşe regretted that she told, "I mean high blood pressure or something," she said. Meral had to get back. "I am looking forward to hearing from you, if you wouldn't mind." "No bother!" said Ayşe, "Sevil is a dear friend for me, you know."

The maidservant was arranged within a week. Two or three weeks passed, and Meral visited her mother again. Her mother was sleeping as usual. This was a good opportunity to talk to the maidservant. "How are you doing; could you get used to the job?" Zeynep was an experienced lady who had similar working experiences in the past. They hired her to assist in cleaning and cooking, but she quickly understood that Sevil was also part of her job. "She won't eat unless I remind her, sleeps any time of the day, and sometimes looks at the television for hours without taking her eyes off. Luckily, she does not need assistance with the bathroom. She usually sits in silence unless someone touches her, but a few days ago, she jumped up from her couch and started uttering meaningless words. Sometimes it felt as if she looked at herself like an enemy." She didn't want to lose the job she had found with difficulty by telling all these right away. In the past, she experienced a similar problem with another family, and they asked her to leave. She was getting by. "No," she said, "I am already accustomed. Sevil is a very good person. We have made friends with one another." Meral felt relaxed. Obviously, her brother was right. She took some time there and left the house for work. "Please call me if anything happens," she strictly cautioned her. "All right," said Zeynep, "don't you worry, I'll call you."

Two more months passed. Meral visited her mother once a week, but she coincided with either her sleeping time or her mom would tell several sentences, tired and inattentive. The house was clean and tidy. Her mother looked well cared but was losing weight. "She has a poor appetite," said Zeynep. "Should we put her on some vitamins?" She tried to find solutions on her own. "Maybe she'll get better; let's wait and see," said Meral.

When she returned home, she still had questions in her mind. Did she receive adequate care? What if she suffers from another disease? If only I could see mom more often, she thought. She remembered her brother, he acted as if everything was all right, but he didn't see his mom for two months. She did the chores, checked Efe's homework, and headed to her bed, tired. She was just about to fall asleep but woke up to the sound of the phone ringing. She heard the voice of a panicked Zeynep on the other side of the phone. "Meral, your mother is lost, she just went out, I cannot find her anywhere," she was crying. "What do you mean lost, where would she go? When did you first notice, didn't she tell you anything?" Questions kept coming but the only sound was crying on the other side of the phone. "All right, I'll be right there, don't worry," she said, putting on some clothes, and left the house. What happened to her mom? Was she abducted? No way, why would they abduct my mom, who would do this? This was something else. Maybe she fell asleep in some part of the house. When she finally arrived there, there were several people in front of the house. One of them was a police officer. She shivered with fear. But did something happen to my mom? As she got closer, she saw her mom looking startled with her nightgown on in front of the crowd. Oh fortunately, her mom was alive. What happened, she inquired and came closer. "We found your mother a few blocks away." The shop-keepers knew her, "They called us seeing she acted strangely, and we took her to her home." Meral hugged her mom crying, "Mom what did you do?" she questioned her mom. Her mom stood motionless. She looked at her face but couldn't see any-thing but the face of someone lost. "Let's get into our home; thank you all," she addressed the crowd. When they got into the home, Zeynep was crying. "I knew this would happen but I thought she would not move away from my sight. I stopped her on previous occasions." Meral couldn't believe what she was hearing. "But how, did this happen before?" "Yes," said the maidservant, "but I could convince her. She all of a sudden wanted to go out, saying there was someone outside, mention-ing names of people who were not there. I didn't tell you considering this would make you sad. She kept blaming me for stealing her money but I knew she didn't do this on pur-pose, so I was patient. She fell on several occasions but wasn't injured. She already walks stonily. Yet again, she doesn't talk much; she eats when I cook and won't ask when I don't. Sometimes she doesn't remember me, asking me whether I am the daughter of a certain person. Why are you here, she asks; at other times, she asks me to take her home. I tell her this is your home auntie, which makes her angrier, so she tries to go out. She often mentions the name of her deceased hus-band. On one occasion, she called the janitor with her hus-band's name; the janitor smiled and went back." Meral listened to her with grief. "Well, are her bathroom habits okay?" "Not too much," replied Zeynep. "Sometimes she messes her clothes but I do what I have to. In the end, we will all get older."

Meral kind of understood what was happening. She thought this cannot be explained simply by old age. Many other elderly people are living active lives on their own, need-ing nobody. "We have to rush to the doctor tomorrow," she said to Zeynep. "I saw a film telling a story of a disease simi-lar to her condition. The woman was just like my mom."

"Okay, I will get Sevil ready tomorrow, don't worry," she said. Meral decided to stay at her mother's that day. She called home to let them know. She also called her brother for tomorrow's arrangements. This time her brother was worried too.

The next day, they dressed up Sevil and took her out. "Where are you taking me? Ahmet is still sleeping," she kept saying. It was more than ten years since she lost her husband Ahmet. "Okay mom, he will be coming," so they could hardly convinced Sevil. When they arrived at the hospital, Sevil first felt uncomfortable. In fact, Meral was more uncomfortable. They didn't know what awaited them. They had an appointment with the neurology clinic. It wasn't easy to control Sevil until they were let in. She would sleep where she was sitting, silently check around when she woke up, and she would sit up and try to go out. Meral convinced her on every occasion telling, "Okay mom sit down, we will now see the doctor." Sevil seemed to quit after several attempts. She suddenly fell asleep, woke up, and started yelling, pointing at somewhere over her head with her hands. "They are there; they came again," she looked in fear. Meral couldn't wait more, and with permission from others in the queue, she got into the doctor's room. "My mom," she said, "she is very bad, like crazy, could you please see her before other patients?" There was a patient and his family in the room. First they couldn't make any sense, but then, in the face of Meral's helplessness, they consented, "Okay you can take your patient in. Our patient is not an emergency." Meral held her mom's arm and took her in. Her brother was outside. The doctor started a long conversation with Meral and asked plenty of questions to her. At the end of the questioning, Meral noticed how many things she skipped and did not notice. She looked at the doctor with a sense of guilt and helplessness. The doctor commented on her mother's condition, telling her what could be done. He said this process had a natural course but certain methods of treatment could be of help. Meral's mind was stuck on the words she heard when the doctor was talking about the diagnosis: Alzheimer's disease, dementia... She thought this would be the case for others. It was surprising to see the disease in someone who was very close…

"Okay," said Meral, "well, we will do what we have to do."

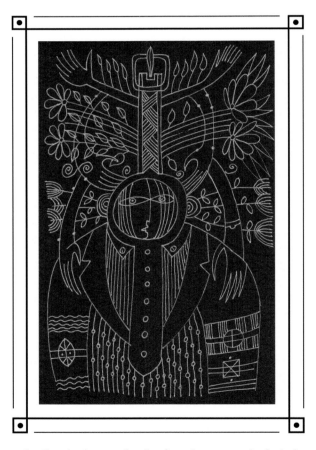

FIGURE 6.1 Inspirations and reflections from neurological phenomena (Image courtesy and copyright of Assoc. Prof. Lale Avşar, Selcuk University School of Art and Design, Turkey. Used with permission)

Chapter 7
Guillain–Barré Syndrome

Gamze noticed that she felt very exhausted when she woke up in the morning. Normally, she was very agile and active lady for her age. She thought "This could be because yesterday was an exceptionally busy day," and got up from bed without giving it a careful thought. Yes, she was lacking in strength, particularly in her legs, for several days. She did not walk much but she thought the housework was tiring. She briefly checked herself, she had almost no fever, but she was feeling feverish. She realized that she was sweating at times.

She got up and finished her bathroom routine before getting the breakfast ready. She could hardly get herself to the kitchen. Her children wouldn't go to school without breakfast. She felt as if she was shuttling between the kitchen bench and the fridge spending twice as much time with her legs heavier with each step. She plopped onto the chair after she finished preparing the breakfast. She had pain in the waist and back, and it was as if the pain went all the way down her back through the spine, wrapping all around her stomach like a belt. It was nothing like diarrhea. She again attributed it to fatigue. It was a permanent pain, and bending and standing were of no good. She assumed that her condition would get better and started caring for her children who knew that the breakfast was ready judging from the noises in the kitchen.

Ş. Öztürk, *Neurological Disorders in Clinical Practice:*
Case Histories for Medical Students and Residents,
In Clinical Practice, DOI 10.1007/978-3-319-23168-6_7,
© Springer International Publishing Switzerland 2016

Her youngest daughter was the most sensitive one. "Hey mommy, you look pale," she said. "Nothing sweetie, just a little tired," she slurred. She thought her daughter could be right when she said, "Mom, you just couldn't shake the flu." She got the flu about 2 weeks ago. As always, she got over the flu within 2 or 3 days without even having to stay in bed. In fact, she was fine until a few days ago but if only this back and waist pain as well as the weakness in her legs were gone. She did the chores without letting the children notice. After seeing them off and shutting the door, she lay on the couch in the living room, "I'll be fine if I get some rest." These thoughts ran through her mind. She felt more exhausted as she lay on the couch. She didn't remember when she last took a vacation. She recalled her mother. She too would keep whining about fatigue. Everyone has a season, she thought, falling asleep. Only minutes later, she woke up with the pain in her back and waist. The house was in full silence as she opened her eyes. At least 1 or 2 hours must have passed. She struggled to sit up. It was even harder this time. She stood up climbing off the couch and headed to the bathroom to wash her face. She really had difficulty walking. The distance between the living room and the bathroom seemed miles away. When she finally got to the bathroom, she laid herself against the corner cabinet, took the toothbrush, and put some toothpaste on it. Her arms were also kind of weak but she could move them. She made an effort to open her mouth to brush her teeth, but her mouth just wouldn't open wide. She tried to smile at the mirror, but to no avail. The muscles around her mouth were virtually frozen. She couldn't explain the situation and, kept brushing, and washed her face and when she at last finished with it, soap was getting in her eyes. She noticed that she couldn't fully close her eyes. Suddenly she was worried. All accounts of paralysis she has heard of and knew attacked her mind. Had Aunt Humay suffered the same thing? No, she had it in only one side of her body. Uncle Ahmet was another example. First he lost his speech, and then he passed away in 3 days. The neighbor's daughter too had facial paralysis but only on one side, but she recovered within several weeks. She had heard of no accounts that were similar to what she was going through. Now, she had to do something. She headed to the telephone with difficulty. Her sister was a clever woman. She would immediately work out a solution. When she told her about her condition, first she got a scolding for a few minutes for her negligence, and then she said she would be there in a moment. She had nothing to do but sit and wait. The doorbell rang several hours later. More's the pity, she was not strong enough to stand up and open the door. Her sister had the keys. She rang the doorbell but after several attempts she opened the door with the key. Her sister was half-sitting on the couch. Her face reflected her awful pain. She made jokes just to relax her sister, but she received no reactions. "she said, why the long face?" "No," Gamze replied. "I cannot move my face." Looking more carefully, her sister too noticed the difference. The area around her mouth and eyes was like a mask. Come on, eat something and I'll take you to the hospital. She hurried into the kitchen and came back with some light stuff. Gamze knew that she had to eat although she never wanted to eat. "You have to eat to survive," her sister said and added some meal. Gamze had a bite but could hardly chew it. She held the food in her mouth, trying to swallow it. The bite was almost stuck there. She just couldn't swallow it. "Swallow it with some water," her sister said passing a glass of water, and she sipped with difficulty. The water went down her trachea accidentally. She began to cough, and her sister was more worried as her face turned slightly purple. "Okay," she said. "Let's not push it. We must go to the hospital." Calling a taxi would do little. So she called an ambulance. After a quick examination, the paramedics concluded that she could need intensive care and some blood tests, and they would look particularly for food poisoning. "Have you eaten canned food," the paramedics asked. "No," said Gamze, "I don't like canned food." "Well, did you experience flu or diarrhea in the last week?" "Yes," Gamze replied, telling her experience with the flu. The emergency team informed Gamze's sister telling that they would ask for neurological consultation. "It could be something important but remain calm. Our colleagues will do their best." The consulting neurologist asked similar questions and made a detailed examination. Meanwhile, Gamze was weaker than ever. "We will take her to the intensive care unit," said the neurologists. "We primarily suspect Guillain–Barré, but to be sure, we have to have a lumbar puncture and make electrophysiological examinations. We will quickly plan your treatment. Don't worry, you are not late; hopefully you will recover soon."

While Gamze and her sister were taken to the intensive care unit, they were being slightly relaxed because they had been admitted early. Although they were anxious about the increased pain and weakness, they were filled with hope in their hearts.

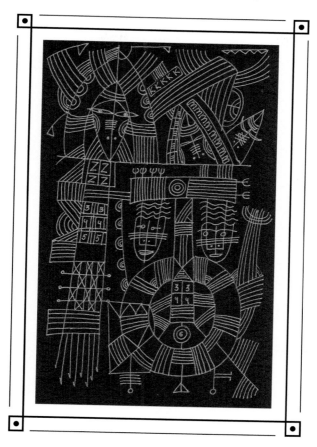

FIGURE 7.1 Inspirations and reflections from neurological phenomena (Image courtesy and copyright of Assoc. Prof. Lale Avşar, Selcuk University School of Art and Design, Turkey. Used with permission)

Chapter 8
Subarachnoid Hemorrhage

Sezgin was in fact a calm, hardworking computer technician who got on well with his office mates. He was 35 but looked as if he was 45. It was really difficulty to annoy him, but when he was annoyed, he became someone totally different. His face became red; the veins in his forehead became more prominent and you would think they would explode. Yet, he did not yell and shout. Only, he constrained himself, and until his anger abated, either stayed in the room or if possible went out and took a quick walk. When he came back, everything turned to its normal course. Occasionally, he held his head between his hands and felt as if everything had stopped. When his colleagues asked if his headache had recurred, he replied indifferently, "Don't worry, I think I am tired that's all." Indeed, a few days later, he would feel relieved. Egemen, the office manager, was not very happy about his situation. He would say to him, "Son, this is headache; you need to take it seriously. At least, go and get your blood pressure taken." While he was saying this, he suddenly remembered his wife's brother who had died suddenly last year. He, too, had complained about his head after a session at the gym and then collapsed all of a sudden. They had taken him to the hospital and it had been found that his blood pressure was too high. The doctors had accused the family, asking, "Haven't you ever thought of having it checked?" But his wife's brother

Ş. Öztürk, *Neurological Disorders in Clinical Practice:*
Case Histories for Medical Students and Residents,
In Clinical Practice, DOI 10.1007/978-3-319-23168-6_8,
© Springer International Publishing Switzerland 2016

was someone obsessed with health who always did exercise and sometimes even went to extreme in this regard. He never thought that his blood pressure might rise. He believed that everything he did was right. People would say like father, like son. However, he had collapsed all of a sudden, and they had lost him without realizing what the reason for the paralysis was.

Sezgin had been alright during the past few days. Everything had been running smoothly. Nothing that might annoy him had occurred. A headache had started suddenly when he was in the toilet and stopped exerting his strength. I have to solve this constipation problem; every time, I also have a headache, he had thought. He had to eat food with more fiber content. He did not like vegetables at all but what could he do? At least, he would eat them as medicine, he thought. He would go out with his friends for a meal. I will eat some salad, he thought. As soon as noon arrived, the four friends got ready and left the office as they had agreed. The restaurant was not very far; it was within walking distance. It was a small diner but its dishes, especially meat dishes, were delicious. They ordered their dishes immediately and began to sip their drinks while waiting for their dishes. When the food came, they added ample amounts of salt and pepper and began to eat. A little while later, his head began to ache again. A waiter who approached them asked if they wanted anything. They ordered coffee. Almost half an hour passed but the coffees did not arrive. The waiter, who had had been dealing with them diligently, had begun to deal with a large group who had just come and therefore forgotten them. "Waiter, we are being late, where are our coffees?" he called. The waiter did not even bother to look at him. He called him again, this time more loudly. No, the waiter would not care about them. He suddenly got angry. "We are your regular clients. What kind of treatment is this?" he shouted. His face had grown crimson and his veins had got swollen. The people in the new group were now looking at him. He got even more crimson and collapsed screaming, "Oh my head!" He was experiencing the severest headache in his lifetime. It was as if his brain would burst. He felt dizzy and nauseated. His friends had got alarmed and were trying to lay him somewhere flat. He suddenly began to experience convulsions. His eyes had been turned to one side, he had bitten his tongue, and his mouth was bleeding. Although his friends tried to keep him steady, his convulsions lasted about 2 minutes. When they came to an end, the place was like a battleground. The people in the neighboring tables had dispersed and others were watching what was going on in amazement and fear. The one who first got a grip on himself was the owner of the place. He ran for the phone, sent for an ambulance, and gave the address. When he finished his call, he turned Sezgin to his side and checked the inside of his mouth with paper tissue. It was only the tongue that was bleeding. Sezgin's trousers and the ground were wet because he had urinated involuntarily. He put a towel under his head and they began to wait. A medical team who had got off the ambulance that had come within a short time surrounded Sezgin. One was taking his blood pressure, another was taking his pulse, and still another was checking his eyes. One called, "Mr. Sezgin, do you hear us?" Sezgin was moving his arms and legs aimlessly but he could not open his eyes. A terrible headache and dizziness still persisted. It was as though his nape had frozen. The nurse in the team announced his blood pressure as 160/90. She asked the people around if he had had high blood pressure before. They replied in sorrow, "We don't know, but we think he did not know, either. He had never mentioned it. But he often complained of headache." "Okay, we must go to hospital immediately," the team said. "But one of you can come with us." Finally, the team, Sezgin, and a friend headed for the hospital in the ambulance. The people in the restaurant looked behind the ambulance still in amazement. When they reached the nearest hospital, they immediately proceeded to the emergency service. Sezgin was put on the hospital stretcher and taken to the rapid response room to give him his first examination. He was opening his eyes occasionally and looking around in astonishment, and there was a meaningless expression on his face. An emergency service doctor wanted to learn what had happened from his friend. Meanwhile, Sezgin vomited again, and upon this, his examination was sped up. His blood pressure was still high. His pulse was irregular. His nape was still very firm. There were involuntary movements in his arms and legs. Hemorrhage was observed during the ophthalmological examination. He was immediately taken to the tomography unit. Zones of hyperintensity were observed between the curves of the brain. The emergency service doctor who saw the tomography asked for consultation with neurology and neurosurgery. Meanwhile, he completed his efforts to do an lumbar puncture. Lumbar puncture showed hemorrhage in CSF. He centrifuged it. The top section was clear and erythrocytes had settled. Yes, he thought. This is a typical case of SAH (subarachnoid hemorrhage). It had to be examined for aneurysm. Aneurysm was detected in anterior communicating artery as a result of vascular imaging. The patient was referred to the interventional vascular department for vascular intervention.

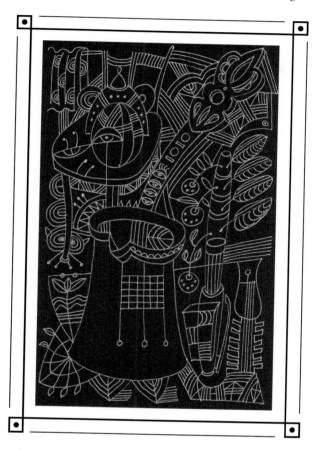

FIGURE 8.1 Inspirations and reflections from neurological phenomena (Image courtesy and copyright of Assoc. Prof. Lale Avşar, Selcuk University School of Art and Design, Turkey. Used with permission)

Chapter 9
Neuropathic Pain

Aysen had not been able to sleep until morning again. Her hands and feet had burned all the time as if there were a fire blazing under them. Even the bedsheets had hurt wherever they had touched. Whenever she told her husband about it, he mocked her saying "Aysen, it is beyond dispute that you are a princess because you are disturbed even by extremely soft bedsheets." She would sigh and say "Only those who suffer know how terrible the pain is. How will you know? You sleep like a log all night." Indeed, these pains had caused her to be bored of life during the past 2–3 years. It had initially begun as if there were pins and needles. It was mostly in her feet but she had started to feel it in her hands, too. Especially at night, her feet felt as though they had been dipped in an ice bucket, and they did not get warm no matter what she did. Therefore, she woke up at night, wore her wool stockings, and slept again. She took them off early in the morning lest her husband saw them and made fun of her. As a matter of fact, the stockings were not of much help and indeed she felt more secure with her ice-cold feet. Sometimes, she had to move her feet all night, getting sometimes in and sometimes out of the blanket, barely making it to the morning. What disturbed her more was the feeling of burning. "What an endless fire is this?" she used to complain. She would rise to her feet, walk out to the balcony, drink cold water, but whatever she did, the

Ş. Öztürk, *Neurological Disorders in Clinical Practice:*
Case Histories for Medical Students and Residents,
In Clinical Practice, DOI 10.1007/978-3-319-23168-6_9,
© Springer International Publishing Switzerland 2016

feeling of burning would not disappear. She took painkillers almost every day. In fact, she had begun take an extra dose which she took before she went to bed at night. There was almost no painkiller that she had not tried. She had tried whatever painkiller she had heard of, on the pretext that it had worked well with the next-door neighbor though she had no information about it. None of the painkillers had relieved Aysen's pains, but she did not give them up lest her pains further increased. She had begun to buy her painkillers directly from the local pharmacy as she was ashamed of seeing the family doctor. When the family doctor had seen her records, she had been very surprised at the list before her. "Hey, what is this Aysen? Your home must look like a pharmacy. You seem to have tried all kinds of painkillers. What do you do with all these drugs?" she asked. "My feet ache and what can I do? I cannot get a decent sleep," she replied in a whisper. The family doctor continued examining the list and asked in the same amazement in her tone, "And there are as many stomach pills here as well. Why them?" "If you had used so many painkillers, your stomach would have been ruined, too. I take them out of necessity; otherwise, stomachache is added to the pains in my feet," Aysen responded defensively.

The family doctor went on looking at Aysen's file. "You have diabetes, don't you? How long have you had it?" she asked. "It has been more than years since my diabetes was diagnosed. My mother also had it. I always feared I would be like her. She used to complain of pains and feelings of burning. And finally what should I see? I have the same complaints. Such is life!" she sighed, while two drops of tears began to trickle down her cheeks.

The family doctor had felt sorry for Aysen's condition. "Hey, don't worry! There is always a cure for anything," she said. Aysen looked incredulously at the young doctor's face. She had visited many doctors but had not been able to find a cure. Could this young and inexperienced doctor find one? All the same, she said, out of kindness, "Thank you doctor, I got used to living like this. My mother had also suffered a lot from this. And so it was my destiny. After all, don't they say 'like mother, like daughter?'"

The young female doctor shook her head in sorrow, "Hey, come on? There is a cure for everything. I can guess the cause of your complaints. You have been suffering from diabetes for years. Diabetics often complain of such conditions."

Aysen looked at the doctor in amazement, "Diabetes? What has diabetes got to do with my feet, Doctor?" My mother also suffered from diabetes and complained of the similar things…she thought, and did not object to the doctor. Was her condition also linked to diabetes? But how?

The doctor was making a phone call in the meantime. She was asking the secretary at the clinic for help to get an appointment with a neurologist. When she ended her speech, she turned to Aysen: "I advise you to see a neurologist as soon as possible. Your diabetes may have affected your nervous system," she said. Just then, the secretary entered the room to tell her about the appointment which she had got for the patient.

The doctor said, "Look, your appointment is ready. I hope that you will have got rid of most of your complaints in our next appointment."

Aysen thanked the doctor and could hardly restrain herself from hugging the young doctor. "Well," she said, "if I get well, then I will make my best cake for you."

The doctor said, "You just get well, that is enough for me. But we will be happy to see you any time," and showed her the way.

Aysen was at the neurology outpatient clinic two days later. She had to wait for a while. She began to talk with the lady next to her. Obviously, she was suffering from the same condition but she did not look so desperate. "I used to be like you, I was trying to get used to my pains and burning, but I learned that it was something that arose as a result of diabetes. All the nerves in my body but especially my feet and hands could be affected by it. I had used so many drugs for years, but all in vain. To my surprise, it appeared to have a cure. The drug a neurologist prescribed me relieved me in a few days. Now, I pay attention to my blood glucose level, too. If blood sugar level follows an unstable course, this condition may increase, they say, which is true in my case. I take care in regard to my diet and drugs and I feel quite alright and I do not miss my follow-ups."

Now, Aysen, too, began to cherish hope. Well, then, she could also get relieved of her pains. She remembered with a feeling of guilt that she had not paid proper attention to her diabetes. She tried to defend herself saying "but these pains rid me of all my joy of life," yet it was in vain. She herself was beginning to feel the reality now. Meanwhile, it was her turn to see the doctor. While she was entering the doctor's room, she smiled, convinced that she would get well.

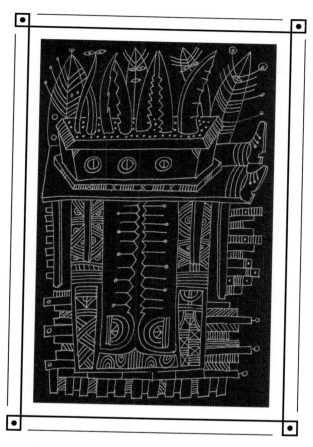

FIGURE 9.1 Inspirations and reflections from neurological phenomena (Image courtesy and copyright of Assoc. Prof. Lale Avşar, Selcuk University School of Art and Design, Turkey. Used with permission)

Chapter 10
Narcolepsy

Aykut had again woken up with nightmares. It was as if he had just avoided death. The situation had been the same for the past few years. Now, he was in fear when the time to go to bed came in case it recurred and he was right indeed. It was something unbearable. Just as he was about to fall asleep or wake up, he felt as if something terrible was coming over him and pushing him down a cliff. Those visions were unspeakable and sometimes so horrible that he did not even want to remember them. In the mornings of such nights, he woke up very unhappy and tired and he did not even want to have breakfast. He just sat there on the bed for minutes and watched the things in the room forlornly. Sometimes, he likened his nightmares to the things in the room like wardrobes and paintings and he had removed some of the articles in the room that he needed thinking that the things he saw before he slept might have affected him. He even gave up watching horror films, which he used to adore, lest they affected his dreams. He took a glance at the clock; it was almost eight o'clock. If he did not get up immediately, he would be late for work again. Recently, his boss had not been treating him well. His friends knew his problems and were trying to handle the situation but his boss was not very understanding. He got up with difficulty and made for the bathroom. He had a quick shower and got dressed but still he felt tired and sleepy.

Ş. Öztürk, *Neurological Disorders in Clinical Practice: Case Histories for Medical Students and Residents*, In Clinical Practice, DOI 10.1007/978-3-319-23168-6_10,

He tried to put the files on the table in order. Since he could not finish some of his work during the day, he had to bring some files home to complete them. At work, he often began to daydream in broad daylight and this of course prevented him from concentrating properly.

He started his car, turned on the radio, but when he opened his eyes, he was still in the garage. He had experienced another detachment. In fact, he had experienced this situation on the way a few more times. Or rather, he had not realized what had happened, but the fact that the place where he was had changed without him being aware of it created doubts in him. Therefore, unless necessary, he had not been using the car for the past few months. But today, there was an important meeting and he had to be on time for it. The boss asked all of them to be present there. He set off without thinking much. When he arrived at his workplace, he found everyone in a hurry for the meeting. He, too, had a file to present. He took a look at it on the computer for the last time, yes, it was alright. He took his computer and files and entered the meeting room. By the time the boss came, everyone was ready. The meeting started. It was a really big project and obviously it was a matter of prestige for the boss to get the project. Aykut was trying to follow the meeting by paying his full attention, but he felt so tired and sleepy that he could not prevent his eyelids from falling occasionally. Eventually, he fell asleep all of a sudden. His head fell before him and he was almost snoring. His friends first looked at him and then at their boss. Finally, the boss called him, "Oh, Mr. Aykut, did you babysit last night? What does this mean?" Aykut opened his eyes upon this and looked around in bewilderment without being aware of where he was. His friends giggled quietly but the boss did not seem to be smiling. Suddenly, everyone got serious. Aykut looked down before him in embarrassment. For quite a while, almost all of his friends had witnessed that he often dozed off at his table, and even fell asleep as soon as he put his spoon in his mouth. They just laughed away, saying "Our sleepy smurf is off again!"

They began to present the files they had prepared one by one. Now, it was Aykut's turn. He promptly went near the presentation screen. What had happened a few minutes ago had extremely embarrassed and excited Aykut. He began his presentation. His boss rose to his feet and asked him to explain the previous slide in a loud voice. His excitement increased further upon this. All of a sudden, he collapsed. He heard and understood the voices around but could not move at all. It was as if his whole body had been paralyzed. He got very afraid. His friends were even more afraid. His boss's face was red all over. It was sure he would be the first person to be blamed if something happened to Aykut. Some offered to bring water while others tried to raise his legs to a higher place. Although Aykut was aware of what was going on, he could not respond in any way. A few minutes later, everything turned to normal. Aykut, who got up, was made to sit on a chair. The whole atmosphere of the meeting had changed now. The boss felt relieved after Aykut had come to. "Go and see a doctor immediately and, if necessary, rest for a while," he said. His best friend was Semih. They left the room together. Semih offered to take him to a doctor immediately but Aykut first wanted to go home. He needed a rest terribly. Semih helped him get into a car and said he would call on him in the evening.

When he came home, Aykut thought over what had happened and concluded that yes they did not look normal at all and decided to go and see a doctor definitely. He turned on the TV and found a football match. His favorite team was not playing but all the same it would do him good to watch the match aimlessly. While he was trying to watch the match, he realized that goals had been scored a few times but he also had missed some.

When evening fell, his friend Semih arrived as he had promised. He was an unmarried friend of his whose family lived in a remote city. He had a girlfriend but he thought he had to save money for a little longer before he got married. Aykut always envied him. He had also had some girlfriends before, but each time they had separated for trivial reasons or both parties had not made enough effort to keep the relationship going. Aykut was feeble and tired in the daytime and uneasy at night. He thought that no girl would bear this kind of lifestyle and so deemed it unnecessary to make an extra effort.

Semih had also brought something to eat. They were convenience foods. They put them on plates and sat in front of the TV. They watched TV until late at night. Semih was delighted to see that his friend was better. It was very late when the match ended. Aykut turned to Semih and said, "If you like, stay here. Don't worry; you will have a good night's sleep on the couch. Where can you go at this late hour?" This sounded reasonable to Semih. There was a comfortable couch in the living room. He retired to the bedroom and they both turned off the lights to sleep. Aykut had not closed his door completely because he was a little apprehensive after what had happened during the day.

Semih had difficulty getting to sleep in this strange room. The snores coming from his friend's room indicated that his friend had fallen asleep immediately. It was odd that Aykut snored so much. It stopped for some time. He wondered why and had a look at him through the door. His friend was not breathing. He got alarmed and rushed to his side instantly. Yes, he was not breathing. He did not know what to do for a while. Right at that moment, Aykut began to breathe again. Semih was now really in doubt as to whether this situation was normal or not. He returned to the living room. He decided to tell him about the situation and urge him to see a doctor. In the morning, when Aykut woke up, he did not seem to be one who had slept well and refreshed. Semih urged him to go to hospital even without having breakfast. Now, Aykut felt he had to consent.

There was a hospital with which their firm was working under contract. When they arrived there, they spoke to a female doctor working at the reception. She said they would consult a neurologist. The neurologist came and they told him the situation in detail. The doctor said they would examine him in the sleeping unit and then asked them to make the necessary arrangements for an appointment. "What will you investigate first?" asked Aykut. The doctor replied confidently, "Narcolepsy!"

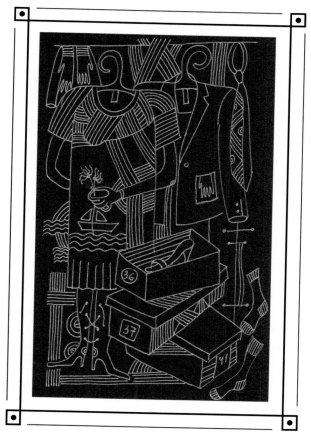

FIGURE 10.1 Inspirations and reflections from neurological phenomena (Image courtesy and copyright of Assoc. Prof. Lale Avşar, Selcuk University School of Art and Design, Turkey. Used with permission)

Chapter 11
Encephalitis

Merih woke up very weak that day. He did not even want to move his hand. He had not been able to recover during the past 15 days. He thought that it had lasted too long. He had a slight temperature and a strange pain had begun in his nape during the past few days. The pain became more pronounced when he moved his neck especially when he had to bend it down. He thought perhaps his neck had been exposed to cold and cramped. Now and then, his head began to spin and felt as if he did not know where he was going. A feeling of sleepiness was coming over him during the day more often. If they let him, he would sleep immediately. He stayed in a dormitory and his roommate complained of his situation. He had not taken part in any activity in the past few days and he did not eat no matter how much his roommate insisted. Even his complexion looked paler in the mirror. He would still be sleeping when cleaning personnel came to clean the room. At first, they did not want to disturb him, but in the end, they could no longer bear it and told him to leave the room or they would be warned by the administration on the grounds that they had not cleaned the room. He rose to his feet with difficulty and went to the canteen. A few of his classmates sitting there said, somewhat sarcastically, "Look, who is coming? So, it means everyone may skip classes then," and laughed among themselves. Merih did not want to see anyone. He

Ş. Öztürk, *Neurological Disorders in Clinical Practice:*
Case Histories for Medical Students and Residents,
In Clinical Practice, DOI 10.1007/978-3-319-23168-6_11,
© Springer International Publishing Switzerland 2016

made for the farthest table so as to be alone. Everything, including the lights, the voices and sounds, and smells disturbed him. He put his head on his handbag and began to sleep as soon as he sat at the table. After some time, during which he did not move at all, the other students realized that there was something wrong. They called him from a distance, but when they could not get any response, they came near him and began to tease him again saying "Hey, you seem to have drunk excessive alcohol last night. Those who are not used to it must not drink such things." Among those students was a girl called Ayla. She was a sensitive and careful young girl. Though Merih was not one of her type, he was one of the students she liked because of his kind and stable behavior. When she took a closer look, she noticed the twitches at the corner of Merih's mouth. She said, "Hey, wait a second. There is something strange with Merih. Look, there are twitches in his face," and pointed at his face. Ediz strained his arm and said, "What of it? My arm is twitching as well, look." Ayla looked at Ediz with disgust. She thought to herself how she had been dating such a boy for 6 months. "Don't make fun, Ediz. Don't you see, he is really twitching and contracting. What if it is something important?"

Suddenly, the others also grew serious. It looked as if twitches had increased further. They gathered around him, unable to decide what to do about it. Merih looked at her but seemed not to see them. They grew more anxious. "It is best if we called one of the professors," said Ayla. We may have to take him to hospital.

The two hurried towards the corridor where the professors' offices were located. They entered the first office they found and said in a hurry "Sir, there is something strange with a friend of ours. We need to take him to hospital but we do not know how to go about it." The professor did not initially realize the gravity of the situation. He said sarcastically, "Indeed, all of you are more or less strange," and chuckled. But when he noticed that the students were serious, he, too, got hurried and called the students' affairs office and asked for help. He was relieved when he learned that an ambulance would arrive soon. Meanwhile, Merih seemed to have got much worse. He was sweating heavily when the ambulance came. "One of you must come with us and give us information," said an ambulance official. All of them looked at one another. Who could go? "I have an exam," said Ediz. The others did not look much willing either. Ayla made for the ambulance, saying, "I am coming." Ahmet looked at Ayla with anger in his eyes. "What has it got to do with you, ha?" he thought.

It was the first time Ayla had seen the interior of an ambulance. It looked like a small hospital: hanging monitors, displays, masks, and oxygen bottles. Merih was lying motionlessly on the stretcher. "Poor child," murmured Ayla to herself. If only his family were with him now. But none of his family was close to Merih. None of the few close friends he had were anywhere to be seen. Merih woke up and muttered incoherent things, made some movements as if pushing away something in the air, and then fell back to sleep again. Ayla began to feel afraid. She wanted to go to the hospital immediately and then from there to school again but the road to the hospital seemed to grow longer and longer. At last, the ambulance came to a halt in front of the emergency department. The attendants rushing there placed Merih on a stretcher and asked Ayla, "Are you a relative of the patient?" Though she replied, "No, I am just a schoolmate," the attendants took her to the doctor's office alongside the stretcher. The emergency department resembled a huge corridor. There were patients' beds on the sides, while intern medical students, nurses, and patients' relatives were running here and there in a hurry. All of a sudden, she felt very awkward. "What am I doing in here," she thought. Meanwhile, Merih had begun to convulse and twitch again. He held his arm hanging down the stretcher in panic. He seemed to have a temperature and he was also sweating. An intern doctor who came near them was trying to fill in a form. "Who is the patient's relative?" he asked. Ayla came to the fore out of desperation. "I am. I am his schoolmate. He got worse at school and we brought him here." "Is your friend a student?" he asked. This was followed by other questions. A female doctor who came to examine the patient and looked more experienced wanted to see Ayla privately. Ayla now really regretted coming there but nothing could be done anymore. The doctor stared at Ayla's face, as if seeking a clue. Finally, she asked the real question. "You said you were a friend. How close were you?" This question surprised Ayla. "Not close. We were only schoolmates. When he got sick, we were in the canteen near him."

The doctor was browsing through the file in her hand, upset by the fact that she had lost a source of information. "Did your friend use alcohol habitually?" she asked. "No, I don't think so," replied Ayla. She would see Merih from afar but she had never seen him intoxicated. He was always sober, and in fact he looked overly serious. The doctor was not to be convinced by this. "Please, be more directly with me," said she, "Are there students using drugs in your school? Have you ever heard about it?" Now, Ayla realized. They would attribute Merih's illness to another cause. "No," she said. "He was weak and he had a temperature. There were contractions and twitches in his face." She noticed that the doctor had got further excited. "All of these symptoms could be because of medicine or drugs or when alcohol use is ended. We need to be sure." In the meantime, one of the intern doctors came running and said, "The patient is having a seizure, sir!" In no time, the doctor rose to her feet and hurried towards where Merih was lying. Merih was in stronger convulsions now. He foamed at the mouth. Ayla felt really afraid. "Let's send for the neurologist immediately," shouted the emergency doctor. They had turned Merih to his side and were trying to clear the foam so that it would not prevent him from breathing. In the meantime, a nurse came near with a syringe in her hand containing medicine intended to stop the seizure. The contractions stopped 5 minutes later. Another nurse announced, "His temperature is 38." "We need to have a consultation with a doctor from the infectious diseases department. Will you phone them, please?" the doctor asked.

Meanwhile, a neurologist had arrived and was trying to understand what was happening. When he learned that the patient was a student, he asked questions similar to the ones asked by the previous doctor. He was more interested in the way the seizure occurred. Were there such contractions before? Was he on a drug? Was he known to have a history of an illness like diabetes? It was impossible for Ayla to answer questions like these. "Let's find a way to inform his family," she said to the doctor. She added, "I know he stays at the dormitory and they must have his address there." The doctor was now persuaded. "Right," he said, "Let's immediately call the dormitory where he stays."

In the meantime, the neurologist had completed his examination of the patient. He said, "I think the patient is suffering from an infection. We had better get the view of the infectious diseases department." Then, he dictated the tests he demanded to an intern doctor. "First of all, let's get a cranial MR; we need to get an EEG taken, too. His seizure may recur. We will need to contact the infectious diseases department and get a lumbar puncture, but the patient is still unconscious and he has no relatives around either." "But this is an emergency and you can make the decision," said the emergency doctor.

"You are right. In that case, we will need to decide on the most beneficial and necessary intervention for the patient," said the neurologist, in agreement with him.

They took Merih to the MR unit immediately. The images indicated that there was nothing to contraendicated for a lumbar puncture, but there were not enough clues as to the presence of an infection. Lumbar puncture was now inevitable and then an EEG was to be taken.

In the meantime, a bed had been prepared for him in the neurology department and Merih was sent there, accompanied by nurses.

The next day, Merih's father and mother had come to the hospital and were anxious while they were talking to the doctor. The neurologist was trying to calm down the parents on the one hand and making explanations on the other.

"Encephalitis is in fact a disease that may do immense harm if it is not treated at an early stage, but fortunately your son was brought just in time. The girl who was with him yesterday was of great help. Without her, our job would have been very difficult. Your son owes his life partly to her."

Ayla, who had just arrived there, had also heard the talk. The fact that the things she suffered yesterday had worked well made her forget all her exhaustion and troubles. Moreover, she noticed that she really wanted to see Merih without delay.

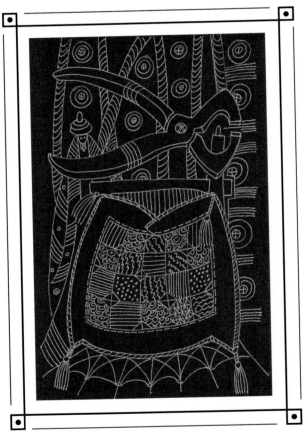

FIGURE 11.1 Inspirations and reflections from neurological phenomena (Image courtesy and copyright of Assoc. Prof. Lale Avşar, Selcuk University School of Art and Design, Turkey. Used with permission)

Chapter 12
Brain Tumors

Deniz had caused the meeting to end in extreme tension, as he had been doing recently. He was the department head of a large advertising firm. He was known for his painstaking attitude in his job, but at the same time he was very popular at work due to his gentle manners and patience towards the employees. As a prominent advertising firm, they usually worked for large campaigns. There were times when they undertook various jobs at the same time and at such times everyone would try to do their best and sometimes they would work until morning. While young staff members usually performed shootings and field work, planning and administration were conducted by more experienced and middle-aged executives like Deniz. Serving as an executive required experience and patience, but fortunately, recruitment of people for such positions was conducted very carefully and often decisions were taken about attendance and performance was evaluated constantly.

When Deniz first started his job, he was 26 years old, and after he had worked for a few small firms, an executive from this firm who he was acquainted with discovered his competence and ensured that he was hired. Since he began to work here, he had completed every task he had assumed fastidiously, be it a small or a big one, and had always been successful. This attitude of his had served as a model for the young

Ş. Öztürk, *Neurological Disorders in Clinical Practice:
Case Histories for Medical Students and Residents*,
In Clinical Practice, DOI 10.1007/978-3-319-23168-6_12,
© Springer International Publishing Switzerland 2016

people around him, and there had always been a meticulous and enthusiastic team working with him. Today, they were working as a team on a project they had undertaken. Deniz was a little absentminded today as he had been in recent months. His friends attributed this to his working hard and implied at every opportunity that he should go on a holiday, but he did not seem to have taken heed of them. He interrupted the presentation prepared by one of the promising young team members a few times and asked him to repeat it. This marred the concentration of the group, and the young staff member who was making the presentation had to resume it with some frustration. When the presentation ended, questions began. Deniz said "I have a question," and when he asked his question, everyone looked at one another. The question he asked had been answered several times during the presentation. The young man who had made the presentation tried to answer saying, "Sir, as I said during my presentation…" but Deniz got angry suddenly and began to shout. Everyone was petrified. This was not a manner they expected of him. How could Deniz have changed like that? However, soon, Deniz noticed what he had done and left the room. When he came to his own office he had a slight dizziness. A slight headache which he had been suffering from for days seemed to have intensified. When he sat down in his armchair, he felt his head had grown heavier. Indeed, he thought he had got extremely tired recently. It was time he had a break, he thought.

When he arrived home, he told his wife and daughter that they could go on a holiday next week but at first they did not believe this. They had not gone on holiday together for years. His daughter asked with a smile, "Are you really sure, dad?" There were 4 days before the holiday and he could set the things right. When they sat at the dining table, he felt a feeling of nausea in his stomach before he took his first morsel. This feeling of nausea had occurred repeatedly recently. Sometimes, he thought it had something to do with the meal, but at other times he noticed that it occurred with no reason at all. After he had eaten a little, he moved to the living room to rest. He felt extremely tired. In the meantime, his daughter was making jokes, and having been irritated by them, he rose to his feet to go to bed. When Deniz retired to the bedroom, his daughter told her mother in a complaining tone, "Dad is getting really unbearable, do you notice that?" "No, don't you see he is very tired. He will get well after the holiday," she replied but she, too, was aware of the recent changes in Deniz's temperament. The gentle and considerate man she had married had begun to turn into one who was rude and furious and did inappropriate things; she wished it would be temporary.

Days elapsed and their holiday had come. They loaded their belongings onto their car. Deniz was an amusing driver. He would make jokes on the way and entertain them. He would find the roads he was driving along for the first time, but this time things were different. Several times, Deniz had taken the wrong road and each time he grew angry and began to shout at the people in the street. His wife started to say, "If only we had flown." They arrived at their destination after a few stops on the way.

Nobody objected when Deniz went to bed, saying "I will sleep for a while." Obviously, they would rather he slept than shouted like that. They rushed to the sea nearby.

When they entered the room in the evening, Deniz was still sleeping. His wife grew worried and said, "Deniz, it is almost evening. Come on, wake up. Let's eat something. You must have already slept enough." Deniz, who could barely open his eyes, held his head and moaned, "I have a terrible headache."

"Come on, get up, then you will feel better." His wife said. He got up but he was staggering when he began to walk. "Did you drink something before you slept in this heat?" she asked seriously concerned.

"No, you know, I fell asleep immediately." At the same time, he was trying to walk holding to the wall. His wife, too, helped him and they were able to get out. When he sat at the table in the garden, he felt a little better. He thought it would be a good idea to drink something and relax a bit before dinner.

His wife objected saying, "You already have had nausea for some time. Why don't you eat something first?" He replied, "I have nothing. I am sure a drink will do me good," and asked for a glass of wine. Then, a second and a third glass came and now his speech started to be inconsistent.

When the dishes came, they were already very hungry. Hardly had Deniz pulled his plate before him when he began to struggle in convulsions. His wife, who was watching her husband in terror and amazement, could not prevent him from sliding down the chair under the influence of convulsions. His eyes had turned to one side and foam came out of his mouth, while wheezing sounds were coming from his throat. His face began to turn black. Several people rushed to his wife, who had asked for help, screaming. They tried to lift him off the ground, but they were not able to stop the convulsions. Eventually, convulsions abated and then stopped. Having opened his eyes, Deniz was looking around meaninglessly. At last, he seemed to come round and asked what had happened to him. His wife and daughter were crying. His clothes were wet and dirty. "We need to go to hospital immediately!" said his wife. In the meantime, the owner of the hostel had already sent for an ambulance. "They will be here in ten minutes," he informed them. He was with his wife and daughter in the ambulance now. His daughter had insisted on coming along, and when nobody had succeeded in persuading her to stay there, they had to take her in. The faces of all three were concerned. They had not fully realized what had happened.

When they arrived at the hospital, they were first led to the emergency service. There, Deniz was asked a series of questions. The emergency doctor decided to consult the neurology department. After questioning in detail, the neurologist demanded   blood   tests   and   brain   imaging. Deniz's wife could not believe what they were going through during the questioning, she realized that she had noticed many things but had not yet taken them seriously. Her concern was further increased when they were on the way to the MR unit. While Deniz was in the MR unit, the neurologist was watching the imaging together with radiologists. The worried expression in their faces was increasing with each film.

"There is a frontal mass, highly probably a malignant cerebral tumor. We will have to talk to neurosurgeons," he informed the interns while Deniz's wife overheard him. Brain tumor! She was looking in panic in the face of these words which she heard but could not believe to be true. Well, that was the reason why they had been experiencing so many changes in recent months then. She was surprised by her own inability to take action and what was to follow was further increasing her fear. Suddenly, she felt a hand touching her on the shoulder. It was the neurologist who had conducted the questioning.

"I need to talk to you. Don't worry, we will do our best," he said, smiling. Really? Is there really anything that can be still done? echoed a voice in her mind. She felt a little better now.

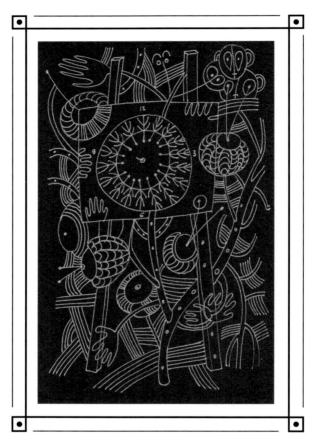

FIGURE 12.1 Inspirations and reflections from neurological phenomena (Image courtesy and copyright of Assoc. Prof. Lale Avşar, Selcuk University School of Art and Design, Turkey. Used with permission)

Chapter 13
Dystonia

Ozan was finally at the interview for the job opportunity which he had been dreaming about so long. Since the day he had decided to study management, managing the international relations of a large firm and opening to the world had been his biggest dream. So far, he had worked in a few small enterprises, but in those businesses, nothing had happened other than a few daily local exchanges of goods. He had heard about this job opportunity via the internet, applied for it, and been invited for an interview together with tens of people waiting outside. The luxurious office where he was reflected the size of the firm. The gentleman opposite him, who he understood to be Mr. Furkan from the name tag on the table, seemed to be one of the leading figures of the firm. As he tried to keep calm, his excitement further increased. All he worried about was the possibility that the spasm in his neck might start again. In recent months, there were involuntary spasms that occurred when he got excited, tired, or angry and caused him to turn his neck to one side. When he first noticed this, he did not take it seriously, thinking that it was because of the cold or that it was because he had slept in an armchair. Since the day he had noticed the situation, he tried to move to his bed as soon as he felt sleepy. Despite all his efforts, the condition got worse when he got excited or angry, especially in the most critical moments. Last week, when he had an

Ş. Öztürk, *Neurological Disorders in Clinical Practice:*
Case Histories for Medical Students and Residents,
In Clinical Practice, DOI 10.1007/978-3-319-23168-6_13,
© Springer International Publishing Switzerland 2016

opportunity to talk to Aynur, a colleague for whom he had developed a liking but had been unable to talk to, that spasm had started again, Aynur's eyes had focused on his neck in amazement. No matter how much he tried to hide the condition, as time passed by, his head had turned to the right rather than to Aynur, who had been sitting opposite him. It was a very painful situation. When his face was contorted in pain, the amazed expression on Aynur's face had turned into one of pity, which had further hurt Ozan. Saying, "I've got to go," he had left there in a hurry. His neck had straightened some time later, but it was too late. As a matter of fact, he had always had difficulty making friends, but this situation had made things more difficult for him. While he was thinking about these things, The director had turned his eyes directly to him and begun to examine him as if he were looking at a painting in an art gallery. Ozan got slightly irritated by this. He had tried to dress as properly as possible before he came here. For a moment, his eyes caught sight of his shoes; "Oh God," he had forgotten to shine his shoes. He had not even noticed it in his hurry in the morning. Now, Mr. Furkan was also looking at his shoes. Suddenly, he felt the spasm in his neck again. "Oh, no, it is back all over again, what shall I do now?" he thought in desperation. The director, who had not even begun to ask his questions yet, was watching the change in Ozan in amazement while trying to start the interview by asking Mr. Ozan, "your name is Ozan, isn't it?" In the meantime, he was holding his neck on the one hand and saying in his hurry to save the day "yes, yes, it is me. Sorry, I have caught cold recently that's why...." At the same time, his hand was fumbling around his neck, seeking a spot to stop the spasm. When he touched below his chin, the spasm got slightly relieved and even disappeared. This had relaxed both Ozan and Mr. Furkan; now, the interview could proceed. He responded one by one to the director's questions, some of which were difficult, required business technique, while others required making comments. He verified the accuracy of his answers sometimes from a smile in Mr. Furkan's face, but sometimes it was impossible to understand anything from the expression on his face, which was now like a competent poker player's. Then, Ozan preferred to rely on his own experiences and continued to say the things he believed were right. When the interview ended, he felt relieved. The director smiled him, "I wish to see you again soon, take care," while shaking his hand. This seemed to augur well for him. He thought it was highly likely that he had got the job. On his way back home, he thought of calling a friend to share his happiness. His friend was at home. He thought it alright when his friend said, "Come to me, we could eat and talk." Therefore, he wanted to go there after buying a cake and cips to eat.

The supermarket was close by. When he maneuvered the car to park it, the spasm in his neck began again. "Again?" he thought in desperation. He became disturbed when his friends saw him in that situation. He waited for a while and when the spasm loosened, he got out of the car and did his shopping hastily. When he arrived at his friend's, he felt rather tired. There was a pain in his neck. They sat at the table immediately. He began to tell his friend what he had experienced quite happily. He did not want to mention the problem he had had about his neck. His friend agreed with him that the meeting seemed to have gone positively. Ozan got excited as he told about the interview. The spasm in his neck began anew. He wanted to talk, one of his hands in his neck, his face in pain, but it was hard. If only I could sleep a little; it will disappear when I sleep, he thought. He knew this from his mother, whom he had visited on holiday. He had made his bed in the living room due to a shortage of space at home and as usual his mother had gone to bed rather late. He was sure that she would frequently pass through his room to go to the kitchen, because she always did so. The next day, she had said, "Son, you must have been extremely tired. You slept like a log, without moving an inch in your bed." He got up in the morning, feeling well, but the spasms during the day caused him to be tired towards the evening.

He spent a few more days, waiting for a reply from the firm he had applied to. Finally, he got the message he had been expecting. They wanted him to come for a trial period next week. When he finished reading the message, he could no longer sit where he was owing to his happiness. He ran to his mother, who was in the kitchen, immediately, and hugged her in jubilation. His mother also hugged him with love, but when she looked at her son, she saw that disturbing spasm in his neck again. Recently, whether he felt sorry or happy, a spasm began in his neck and that handsome son of hers formed a strange picture. On top of that, he was going to start a new job now. She suddenly got worried about her son and tried to persuade him to go to hospital, saying, "Look, sonny, you will start a new job; come, on, do not object to me any more. Let's see a doctor. Maybe, it is something insignificant and you would get cured of it immediately." Ozan wanted to object again, but his mother would not be persuaded. "OK, let's go tomorrow," he said in assent. His mother called the university hospital where she routinely went and asked for an appointment for her son with the neurology clinic. Indeed, she had investigated the matter before and learned that it was the neurology department that dealt with this kind of spasms.

When she hung up, she was relieved because now they had an appointment for tomorrow. When they arrived at the polyclinic, Ozan saw that a few of the people waiting at the door had the same spasms. Interesting, he thought; other people also had the same situation, it seemed. But, what if those patients did not get cured? It might be because of this reason perhaps that they were large in number. When they went in, the doctor met them as if they were familiar. Obviously, he was accustomed to such patients.

After a long period of questions and answers, they moved to the examination couch. Towards the end of the interview, having already got bored and nervous, Ozan's spasm began again.

At the end of the examination, the doctor said to him, "You have dystonia; first, we will try to understand what causes it. Your blood tests and radiological examination will help us. Then, we will plan a treatment for you." Ozan felt slightly relived, having heard that his condition was at least curable, but even as of now, the tests began to seem to him time-consuming and tiring. He looked at his mother accusingly, but she seemed to say in a persuasive expression in her face, "OK, we started and will finish it."

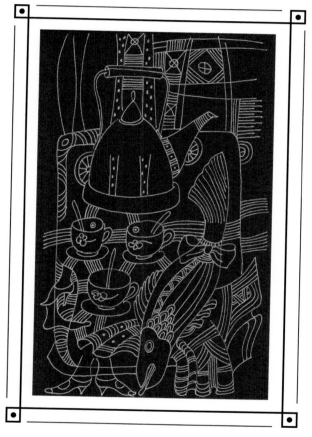

FIGURE 13.1 Inspirations and reflections from neurological phenomena (Image courtesy and copyright of Assoc. Prof. Lale Avşar, Selcuk University School of Art and Design, Turkey. Used with permission)

Chapter 14
Myasthenia Gravis

On her way back from a visit to a friend, she again had difficulty getting on the bus due to exhaustion. Melike had been feeling invariably tired in recent months. Those who had known her before felt this change immediately and initially thought that she was sad and lacked enthusiasm, but when they saw that she found it hard to do things she wanted to do most, they understood that the problem had nothing to do with sadness or depression. Her spouse was the one most affected by this situation. In the past, Melike would wash the laundry and iron and put them away in a single day. However, it was not like that anymore. She had difficulty even standing up, and it took her minutes to remove the bed sheets. She could not hang the wet clothes she had taken out of the washing machine; she hung a few of them, came back, sat and rested, and went again. Mehmet would ask "Do you feel pain, Melike?" "No, it is not pain; I have no strength; I cannot even raise my arms" she would reply each time. He had not heard of such a disease. It seemed as if his wife had changed and become a lazy person. He sometimes asked himself if she was doing that out of obstinacy. We have not been on good terms recently. But why doesn't she talk openly to me? I am the same old me; I haven't changed a bit. Why hasn't she said anything until now and then now suddenly she is behaving like this. As a matter of fact, I am trying to help her. I am

Ş. Öztürk, *Neurological Disorders in Clinical Practice:*
Case Histories for Medical Students and Residents,
In Clinical Practice, DOI 10.1007/978-3-319-23168-6_14,
© Springer International Publishing Switzerland 2016

87

doing all the shopping on the grounds that she can't lift heavy things. I also help with the cooking. What else can I do, he thought.

Their children were also aware of the situation. Their 14-year-old son was in fact happy with the situation because his mother entered his room less often. In the past, his room was full of activity, his mother cleaning the room or taking the laundry. He would always be scolded by his mother for the mess in his room. Now, his mother was not around, there were no warnings, so he was alright. He did not mind the state of the room. On the other hand, their 10-year-old daughter had begun to complain that her hair had not been done properly or her clothes had not been adequately ironed. She had long hair and every morning her hair was combed and made into a plait. Her plaits had become loose and untidy recently. Her mother often would come to school, but she no longer wanted to see her at school. She invariably looked feeble and glum. Her hair was unkempt, there were spots on her face, and it seemed as if her complexion was getting thinner and harder each day.

She felt a little better when she woke up in the morning and looked forward to the day with hope. She thought, "Maybe exhaustion will not come over me today; perhaps it has even gone away."

A few more weeks passed in this manner. One day in the afternoon, her feebleness increased further. Her eyelids began to fall. Indeed, her eyelids seemed to be falling towards the evening, but when she rested, they seemed to get well; but everything recurred soon. She saw the objects on her right double. At first, she made fun of herself, saying "As though I have drunk a bottle of wine." But, the situation was getting more and more serious. Her double sight seemed to be increasing. She decided to wait until evening. When her husband came from work, he had noticed that there was something strange in her look but her dropped eyelids had distracted him and prevented him from asking "Are you tired again, Melike?"

When they sat down at the table for dinner, Melike had difficulty both chewing and swallowing her first morsel. It was the same with the other morsels. She could barely fill her stomach. Although she made an effort not to show her situation, her plate, which was still full, did not escape his attention.

The whole family participated in the task of clearing the table. In the late hours of the evening, Melike even began to find it difficult to breathe. It felt as if something was pushing hard against her chest and made her breathless. When her color started to change, her husband grew anxious. "Melike, your situation is deteriorating, we need to go to the hospital, look, you cannot even breathe, don't object anymore" he said and at the same time rushed to the children's room.

He tried to calm them down saying "I am taking your mother to hospital, she is having difficulty breathing but don't worry, she will be alright."

Melike had found it really hard to get into the car. If only I had sent for an ambulance, he thought, but then he did not like the idea of troubling the neighbors at this late hour of the day.

When they arrived at the emergency service of the nearest hospital, Melike seemed to have gone darker in color. She was put on a stretcher and taken to the emergency intervention ward. While he was watching Melike being taken like this, young doctors who approached him with badges on their chests inscribed "intern doctor" began to ask him questions.

"When had the shortness of breath begun? Had she suffered from another disease before? Was she on any medicine?" As soon as the questions ended, he hurried to his wife. On the one hand, oxygen was being given to her, and on the other hand, her ECG was being recorded. For a moment, he remembered the heart attack he had had 2 years before. They had also given him the test called ECG immediately. But, his wife's situation was not at all similar to what he had experienced. The doctors around were involved in a discussion. A doctor who he understood to be a neurologist was asking Melike some questions and in the meantime checking her pupils, muscular strength, and reflexes.

Let's get an imaging immediately; eye movements are not OK. If we exclude conditions related to brain stem, we need to assess her in terms of myasthenia gravis. The patient may have a myasthenia seizure.

"Myasthenia?" asked Mr. Mehmet, "What do you mean by that? Something like a heart attack?" One of the young doctors touched him on the shoulder and explained. "Don't worry, it is not as dangerous as that, but still it may jeopardize the patient's situation if it is not treated appropriately." And he gave him brief information about myasthenia gravis.

When he looked back on the past, Mehmet understood everything more clearly. All those exhaustions, changes… He regretted his failure to interpret what had been happening to his wife, while looking at his wife, who had been taken to the imaging room.

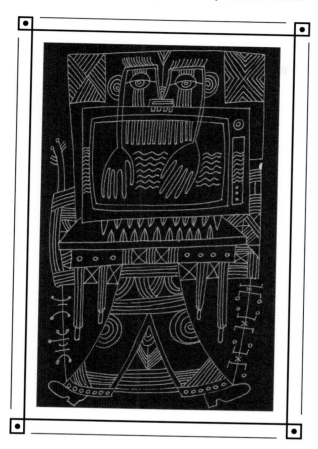

FIGURE 14.1 Inspirations and reflections from neurological phenomena (Image courtesy and copyright of Assoc. Prof. Lale Avşar, Selcuk University School of Art and Design, Turkey. Used with permission)

Chapter 15
Transient Ischemic Attack

Meliha had as usual got up early that morning and began to do the cleaning work at her summer house. She had been working in the garden since morning. Her garden was a source of pride for her. Her daughter, son-in-law, and grandchildren would come on holiday in the afternoon. She would always expect that part of the year to come impatiently. She suddenly remembered her husband. "If only he were alive, too, our grandchildren used to love him so much" she thought, and instantly tears welled from her eyes. She had lost her husband due to a heart attack 3 years ago. They had quite a lot of difficulty having this summer house built so that they could spend their summer holidays pleasurably. Her husband, Mehmet, had been suffering from heart disease for some time and had really spent a huge effort to have this house completed. Unfortunately, they could spend only two summers together in this beautiful house.

She wiped the tears in her eyes and walked towards the house to continue doing her job. There was a lot to do at home. The grandchildren would change the house into a mess in a single day, but anyway she would clean it. She wanted to meet them in a clean and tidy house. After all, she was a woman famous for her cleanliness and fastidiousness. Her neighbors kept teasing her, "Come on, Meliha, why do you spend so much effort on a summer house? After all,

Ş. Öztürk, *Neurological Disorders in Clinical Practice: Case Histories for Medical Students and Residents,* In Clinical Practice, DOI 10.1007/978-3-319-23168-6_15, © Springer International Publishing Switzerland 2016 everywhere is open and it gets dirty soon." Meliha would not take heed of them and keep doing the housework, smiling. Her health seemed to be good, too. Only, she suffered from high blood pressure and tried to take her drugs regularly except when she forgot. I feel capable for the time being. Why shouldn't I do it, she thought and did all her work on her own without asking anybody for help.

The children could come soon. All of a sudden, a feeling of numbness began in her right arm. She could not squeeze the cleaning cloth in her hand adequately. She entered the house, thinking "I think I have got very tired." She sat down on a chair in the kitchen and rested a few minutes. The numbness persisted although 15 min had elapsed. She wanted to get up and wash her face in the bathroom. She thought it would do her good. When she bent down to wash her face, she saw herself in the bathroom mirror. Her face seemed to look awry. It was as if the right corner of her mouth was lower. The groove on the edge of the lip in that corner had almost disappeared and the lines had also decreased. She wanted to look at her teeth, but the right side of her mouth was not contracting and the corner of her mouth was sliding to the left side. She was suddenly alarmed by this. "What is happening to me," she muttered, and it was as if the words were also coming out strangely. She found both her voice and her words odd. She wanted to wash and dry her face quickly. She sat at the nearest table in fear. She could call someone, but she did not dare to get to her feet, fearing that she might fall. She waited almost 10 min not knowing what to do. Then, the numbness in her arm began to subside. She checked her hand by tightening her fist. Not bad, she thought. It was getting better. Instantly, she ran to the mirror and checked her face for a long time. She moved her lips and eyes and saw that they looked normal now. She heaved a sigh of relief, saying, "Fortunately, it is gone!" Her voice had also turned to normal. Thankfully, it was gone before the children came, she thought. She decided not to say anything to the children about it. They will be worried needlessly. They come here on holiday once in a blue moon. Let me not spoil their joy, she thought.

The door bell finally rang. The voice of her naughty grandchild was coming from outside.

She rushed to the door in jubilation. How much she had missed them! Perhaps under the influence of what she had gone through a little while ago, she was hugging them and shedding tears at the same time. Her daughter felt that something out of the ordinary had happened. She tried to calm down her mother, saying "What happened, mum? What are these tears for? See, we are all here." The naughty grandchild interrupted, "Not all of us. Grandpa is not here." Her daughter cast an angry look at her grandchild. Having received the message and noticing the influence of her words, the grandchild headed to the other room in embarrassment. Soon, everything turned to normal. Her daughter was trying to lay the table, Meliha was taking out one by one and putting on the plates the dishes which she had been preparing for 2 days ago and had stored in the fridge. At last, the table was ready and they all sat down at the table. All the dishes were delicious, and Meliha was smiling due to the praises her children were showering on her while at the same time urging them to eat more. This was something she always did, insisting that her guests taste more of her dishes. The children, in their turn, took ample amounts in an effort not to hurt her. Her son-in-law teased her saying, "I will have to start my diet anew, mummy!"

"Come on, one should not go on a diet at your age. You are young. Eat whatever you like. Look, at my age, you cannot eat even if you want to. No salt, no oil, No this No that! So, well then. What will I eat? I haven't eaten a meal full with salt and oil" she complained and at the same time took the salt cellar and began to sprinkle on her plate.

"Alright, alright, mum. Of course, you will have to do so for the sake of your health" said her daughter and touched her on the shoulder. Now, they had made it up again.

Upon the mention of health, Meliha remembered the situation she had experienced a few hours ago. She was in doubt about whether to tell the children or not and finally she decided not to tell again.

After the meal, they all lay down on couches or divans. The journey had tired them.

Meliha, too, looked tired. Both the preparations and the incident she had experienced had really tired her. Her daughter noticed the situation and said, "Mum, I will make coffee for us all so that we will be refreshed!" and headed for the kitchen.

Meliha looked behind her with love, thinking what a nice girl I have raised, how understanding she is!

They watched TV for a little while more and then all retired to their rooms.

In the morning, everyone was woken by the voice of the naughty grandchild. He was hopping and skipping around, shouting before the doors "Come on, let's go to the sea!" They all loved the sea. The son-in-law had engaged in swimming when he was young. Her daughter, on the other hand, had been nicknamed mermaid since her childhood. Wherever she saw the sea, you could not keep her out. However, Meliha was not on good terms with the sea. For her, the sea was a spectacle needed to look at while drinking tea, that's all!

The breakfast was ready when everyone had got up. Meliha had done her best again. The son-in-law tried all on the table, "mum, this is delicious, oh, that is delicious, too." The granddaughter was again in a hurry, "Come on, let's go!" and, indeed, got everyone hurried, too.

While she was preparing the bags for the beach, her daughter called, "Mum, are you ready, too?" Meliha was not feeling well. Her head felt heavy. It was as if a pain originating in the neck was surrounding her head all around. It would be better for her to stay at home and rest. "No, dear! Don't worry about me! After all, I go to the sea every day. You go without me!" Her daughter did not insist much as she knew her mother well enough. "Ok, then! You rest here. We might eat out this evening!" she called out to her.

When they left home, it was as though everywhere had turned to their usual quiet again. If only they were here all the time, Meliha thought. But, life was not like that... everyone had their own life and purpose in life.

I had better tidy up and then take a rest, she thought.

Her headache seemed to have increased. She attributed it to exhaustion again. After dealing with the flowers for a while, she sat down on the chair in the garden and got lost in thought. All of a sudden, that numbness in her right arm began again. "Again!" she thought, with worry. She touched her arm with her other hand. She did not seem to feel it. She opened and closed her hand. It began to get weak. When she remembered what had happened yesterday, she got up and looked at her face. There was nothing unusual in her face, which relieved her a little. "It will pass away soon anyway!" she thought. Right at that moment, she heard the doorbell ring. She rose to her feet to open it, but when she got to the door, she noticed that her hand did not have the strength to turn the key. She was able to unlock it after a long struggle. Her daughter was at the door and looking at her worriedly. "What happened mum? It took you ages to open the door! Ersan left his ball at home, and I came back to pick it. But it seems that it is just as well I came. You don't look well," she said.

Meliha tried to deny again, saying in an effort to calm her down, "No, dear. My arm feels a little numb that's all. It happened yesterday again but passed away soon. Don't worry, it will pass away again!" Her daughter asked with concern in her voice "What! It occurred again yesterday and you didn't tell us? What if it is something serious? Look, it has happened again today. I watched on TV the other day. More serious diseases might underlie such transient loss of strength, they said. Please, don't object, we are going to see a doctor immediately!"

Meliha realized that she could no longer object to her. Her daughter changed her clothes quickly, called her husband to say that she would not return to the beach, that she would go to hospital with her mother but that there was nothing to worry about.

When they arrived at the hospital, they were first directed to the emergency service. There, a doctor who interviewed Meliha asked her detailed questions especially about what had happened the day before. When he combined them with what had happened today, his face grew ever more serious.

Medical examination began immediately after that. First, they took her blood pressure and checked her heart and lungs with a stethoscope. In neurological examination, her right arm was found to be still weak and numb, but it was getting better. When the examination ended, the doctor said to her,

"Mrs. Meliha, your systolic blood pressure is 180, and diastolic is 95; there is loss of strength in your right arm, but even if it is getting less, you had it yesterday, too. You may be experiencing temporary embolisms in your brain vessels. We will consult a neurologist."

When the neurologist came, first he learned about what Meliha had experienced yesterday and today as well as her medical history and the medicines she was on. After he completed his examination, he turned to both the emergency doctor and Meliha and said, " We need to take brain imaging. We need to have CT and MR."

After the imaging was completed, the doctor came near them again. In the meantime, Meliha's complaints had totally disappeared. He said, "Mrs. Meliha, you had a small embolism, but thankfully, the vessel opened immediately and did not leave a permanent effect. However, the situation is very important for us because it may be the precursor of a greater stroke. We have to investigate the factors that might cause this condition and treat them. Don't forget! Transient ischemic attacks are indeed precursors that could protect you from more serious strokes. We need to grasp this message and do what is necessary. It is lucky that you came to hospital immediately."

Meliha looked at her daughter gratefully. Well then, it was important, she thought. Now, she was prepared for whatever to come.

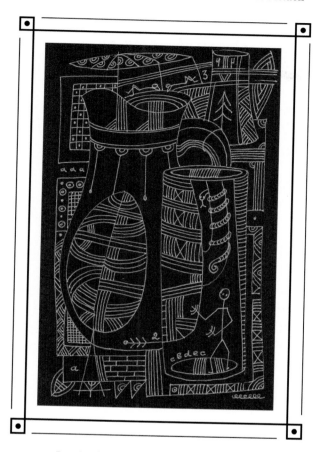

FIGURE 15.1 Inspirations and reflections from neurological phenomena (Image courtesy and copyright of Assoc. Prof. Lale Avşar, Selcuk University School of Art and Design, Turkey. Used with permission)

Chapter 16
Amyotrophic Lateral Sclerosis

When he was leaving the training ground, Arda was thinking about how tired he had become again. He was dispirited again, and it did not elude his friends' eyes while his trainer seemed to be at the end of his tether.

He had wanted to be a footballer since his childhood and finally he had managed to be a member of one of the best teams in the country. His mother kept saying that even when he took his first steps, whenever he saw a ball, he ran towards it and began to play with it. His neighbors still related, snickeringly, the accidents he experienced while he was playing football in his adolescence. Playing football was the reason why he received most of the warnings at school. As soon as the intermission bell rang, he picked up his ball, ran out, and never returned before being warned by his teachers. Everyone had got used to his behaviors of this sort. His friends, especially the girls, admired the tricks he did with the ball! When they were around, he performed his best tricks and almost danced with the ball. He could barely finish school and spent the whole summer at football camps. The trainer of a big football club had seen him at the camp and sent him news via the manager of the camp to recruit him to the youth squad. His parents were middle-class civil servants. They had difficulty making ends meet. Therefore, they wanted Arda to go to university and become an engineer with a high salary, but

Ş. Öztürk, *Neurological Disorders in Clinical Practice:* *Case Histories for Medical Students and Residents*, In Clinical Practice, DOI 10.1007/978-3-319-23168-6_16, © Springer International Publishing Switzerland 2016 they were aware that Arda's tendencies and his study pace would not match their choice. Arda had now become a rather healthy, strong, and agile young boy. He was also very handsome. Whenever his mother looked at him, she saw a prince in him and prayed that his fortunes would be equally good.

When the camp manager informed his parents of the offer made by the football club, they had initially become very anxious. "Could one bring home bread by playing football?" they thought. Yes, they knew that famous footballers were extremely rich, but how many could have that chance? They asked permission to think it over. They would also discuss the matter with Arda. It was impossible not to notice the glimmer in their son's eyes at the mention of the topic. It was obvious that he would greatly enjoy doing that job.

"Look, son" said his father, "Alright, join that team but this is on condition that you also get a university degree."

All of a sudden, Arda was on top of the world. His trainer would most likely help choose an appropriate university for him.

He could choose a department that would not interfere with his football career. His parents had relaxed when he promised to attend university. After that day, Arda had entered a period with a busy schedule. He had trained almost 5–6 h a day and studied for the university examination during the remaining time. Months had passed in this manner, he got a place at university, and this had greatly gladdened the family. In the meantime, his football career had now assumed an ascending turn. He had stood out with his hardworking personality and discipline and become the captain of the team. His next goal was to become a permanent member of the team. He had often played as the striker of the team due to his speed and strength. Years had elapsed in this manner; he had moved up the career ladder fast and got a solid place in the senior team. He had been playing in the same team with an ever-increasing performance for almost 10 years.

He had been leading a comfortable life with the money he had been earning and supporting his parents, too. In fact, he had bought a flat for his mother at a location she had much desired. His age had now reached a period that was about to exceed the best age for football and therefore had to act taking into account his future. He was 36 and it was difficult for him to do this job in his forties. Indeed, he had started to get tired easily recently. He had cramps in his legs in almost every match. When he told his trainer about this, he had initially said it was because he had played without warming up adequately and warned him to be careful in that regard. He never began football matches any more, but the cramps still persisted. This time, his friends said it was because of calcium deficiency, and therefore, he started to consume ample amounts of milk, yoghurt, and cheese. His cramps had not disappeared; instead, twitches had begun in his arms and legs. "These are happening because I am getting very anxious about my future," he thought and tried to relax himself. In fact, once he had even gone to see a psychologist a friend had recommended. He had felt a little at peace on that specific day, but neither cramps nor twitches had stopped. The psychologist's eyes had once lingered on Arda's hands and said "You have such thin hands, like an artist's hands rather than a footballer's." Arda in return had looked at his hands and replied, "Thank you, they did not use to be like this." Indeed, his hands seemed to be getting smaller and thinner gradually. He remembered how difficult it had been for him to open the top of a jar recently. He had thought "I must take some exercise to strengthen my hands." He had not gone to see the doctor again, and instead he had tried to increase his exercises. One day, a cramp that had begun in his leg in a critical position had caused him to lose an opportunity that might have led to a goal. He had begun to encounter such cases more frequently and had to sit in the substitutes' bench. His trainer was a very stern and disciplined person and did not tolerate such situations. At the end of that year, he had been transferred to another team. He was doing his best in this team, which was not as bright as the first one and trying to cope with his cramps, muscular twitches, and weakness that was increasing gradually. He was also making an effort so that people would not notice them. It would be difficult for him to lead his life if he did not work. Unfortunately, his friends who used to be beside him when he earned well were no longer around, and it was hard for him to lead his life in the past standards. Fortunately enough for him, his wife Nihal was a very understanding person and always demonstrated her love for him. On the other hand, tournaments urged him to travel to other cities.

One day, they were travelling on the team's bus and talking loudly. Everyone was given water. He had become very thirsty, so he wanted to drink the water out of the bottle directly rather than wait for the glass. It was something he often did, but this time the water that filled his mouth suddenly flowed into his windpipe and he began to cough wildly as if choking. That day, he tried to quench his thirst with more careful and small sips. This incident began to occur more frequently in the subsequent days. He now also had difficulty swallowing. He wanted to stand in front of the mirror and look into his throat. Meanwhile, his eyes caught sight of his tongue, which he had put out. It felt as though all the fibers were moving freely. It was like small worms were moving alongside one another. Also, his tongue seemed to have become smaller. He thought it was strange but did not give it much thought. There was no redness in his throat. He thought it would disappear soon and therefore tried not to think about it. However, he was trying to be as careful as he could when he drank something. He was taking small morsels and behaving quite slowly, but then he had difficulty finishing his meal in time, and when his friends rose from the table, he had to follow suit. He was also losing weight. His wife had noticed that his clothes had become too big for him and said, "You are working too hard; if only you could relax a bit." Already, his trainer's and his friends' behaviors indicated that he would not stay on the team much longer. That day, he had not performed well again. He had grown short of breath after running a while. It was as if his chest did not allow breathing.

When he came to the team's grounds for training the next morning, he took a few sips from the drink they had distributed but instantly he began to cough. This time, his cough did not stop and his face almost became purple. Everyone got alarmed upon this. They immediately sent for the team's doctor. By the time the doctor arrived, Arda had relaxed a bit but still he looked extremely feeble. After a general examination and checking the lungs, the doctor said, "We need to send him to a better-equipped facility. His lungs do not look fine." His face was an anxious one.

Arda, his trainer, and wife applied to one of the large hospitals of the city. They had deemed it appropriate to start the examination from the chest diseases unit as his lungs were problematic.

A chest disease specialist examined Arda and especially listened to his lungs carefully. "I must see our patient's X-ray and if necessary his tomography." Directed to the radiology unit, Arda and his wife began to think that things were getting increasingly serious. They wanted them to finish as early as possible but at the same time could not help thinking, "Is it already too late?" When they showed the X-ray to the chest diseases specialist, the doctor said in a desperate manner, "Your problem is not in your lungs. There might be a problem with your breathing muscles; therefore, I will refer you to the neurology department." They got an appointment with the neurology polyclinic. The trainer got alarmed as soon as he heard this news, thinking "What a situation! If it is a neurological problem, then there will be a problem with the games." They went to the neurology outpatient clinic together. The neurologist talked to Arda in detail. When he completed his examination, he demanded an EMG of the patient.

While he was heading for the EMG unit, Arda looked at the demand form and saw the word; Amyotrophic Lateral Sclerosis?

Dupuytren's Contracture

Marco Rizzo
Editor

Dupuytren's Contracture

A Clinical Casebook

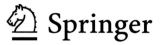 Springer

Editor
Marco Rizzo, MD
Professor, Department of Orthopedic Surgery
Chair, Division of Hand Surgery
Mayo Clinic
Rochester, MN, USA

ISBN 978-3-319-23840-1   ISBN 978-3-319-23841-8   (eBook)
DOI 10.1007/978-3-319-23841-8

Library of Congress Control Number: 2016943432

Printed on acid-free paper

This Springer imprint is published by Springer Nature
The registered company is Springer International Publishing AG Switzerland

Preface

Dupuytren's contracture is a disease of the fascia. This genetic condition tends to affect persons of northern European ancestry, with predominance in men. Most patients seek intervention when their motion is compromised enough to affect function. There is no known cure and recurrence is a constant concern.

Over the last 10–15 years, multiple treatment options for the management of Dupuytren's have come to light. Both office-based and surgical management are available. We are pleased to offer this textbook highlighting the current treatment options for this often challenging disease.

The format of this textbook is case-based. Through the use of individual cases, the authors have highlighted the presentation, indications, technical aspects/pearls, outcomes of treatment, and conclude with a brief discussion. We hope that the book will be a reliable quick reference for the various clinical presentations of Dupuytren's contracture and their treatments. It is my hope that this book will be an excellent resource for surgeons of all levels of experience.

The table of contents highlights the spectrum of treatment options for Dupuytren's disease. The initial chapters discuss nonoperative treatments ranging from orthosis/tissue mobilization, corticosteroid injections, needle aponeurotomy and collagenase injections. Various surgical interventions/techniques follow including: fasciotomy, fasciectomy, open palm, and dermatofasciectomy. Treatment of recurrent disease and its special considerations are also discussed. Chapters discussing the use of skin grafting, illustrating the special challenges associated with revision surgery, and "end of the line" interventions such as arthrodesis and amputation are also included. Less common aspects of Dupuytren's are reviewed as well. Case vignettes that address treatment and special consideration in younger patients, the role/use of dynamic external fixators in Dupuytren's care, correction of distal interphalangeal (DIP) joint contractures and treatment of dorsal finger (Garrod's) nodes round out the chapters of the textbook.

There are many persons to thank for making this book a reality. I am greatly indebted to all the authors for their generosity in providing the chapters. I sincerely appreciate the sacrifice from their busy schedules to share their expertise and experience and to give selflessly. I learned so much from all of them and know that the reader will agree. I cannot thank you enough.

I also am most grateful to all the staff at Springer including Patrick Carr and Kristopher Spring as well as Ms. Hemachandrane Sarumathi and everyone as SPI Global. Their guidance through this process from its inception through completion has helped make this experience a joy rather than chore. I remain indebted to their generosity.

Finally, I am eternally grateful to my family: Hope (my wife) and Hope (my daughter), whom I love dearly. While I do not acknowledge it enough, I sincerely appreciate their love, sacrifice and continued support of my academic endeavors. They remain the greatest inspiration and joy of my life. "When you love someone, you see them the way God intended them to be." – Fyodor Dostoyevsky.

Rochester, MN, USA   Marco Rizzo, MD

The original version of this book was revised. An erratum to this book can be found at DOI 10.1007/978-3-319-23841-8_20

Contents

Contributors

Jonathan P.A. Bellity, MD Department of Hand Surgery & Peripheral Nerve Surgery, Royal North Shore Hospital, University of Sydney, St. Leonards, NSW, Australia

Prosper Benhaim, MD Department of Orthopedics, Division of Plastic Surgery, University of California–Los Angeles, Los Angeles, CA, USA

Paul Binhammer, MD, FRCS(C) Hand Wrist and Microvascular Surgery, Sunnybrook Health Sciences Centre, Toronto, ON, Canada

M.S.K. Bismil, MBBS, MS, FRCSEd, DLM The World Wide Awake Hand Surgery Group, Queen Anne Street Medical Centre, London, UK

Quamar M.K. Bismil, MBChB, MRCS DipSEM MFSEM DMSMed FRCSEd The World Wide Awake Hand Surgery Group, Queen Anne Street Medical Centre, London, UK

Atanu Biswas, MD, MS Mayo Clinic Hospital, Phoenix, AZ, USA

John S.D. Davidson, MD, FRCSC Division of Plastic Surgery, Hotel Dieu Hospital, Kingston, ON, Canada

Nathan Douglass, MD Department of Orthopedic Surgery, Stanford University Medical Center, Redwood City, CA, USA

Reid W. Draeger, MD Department of Orthopaedics, School of Medicine, University of North Carolina, Chapel Hill, NC, USA

C. Liam Dwyer, MD Department of Orthopaedic Surgery, UPMC-Hamot, Erie, PA, USA

Jan-Ragnar Haugstvedt, MD, PhD Department of Orthopedics, Østfold Hospital Trust, Moss, Norway

Ali Izadpanah, MD, FRCSC Department of Plastic Surgery, Centre Hospitalie de l'Universite de Montreal, Montreal, QC, Canada

Sidney M. Jacoby, MD Department of Orthopaedic Surgery, Thomas Jefferson University Hospital, The Philadelphia Hand Center, PC, Philadelphia, PA, USA

Elizabeth O. Johnson, PhD Department of Anatomy, School of Medicine, National & Kapodistrian University of Athens, Athens, Greece

Karsten Knobloch, MD, PhD, FACS SportPraxis, Hannover, Germany

Zinon Kokkalis, MD Department of Orthopaedics, School of Medicine, University of Patras, Patras, Greece

Juliana Larocerie-Salgado, MSc, OT Reg (Ont) Department of Hand Therapy, Roth-McFarlane Hand and Upper Limb Centre, St. Joseph's Health Care Centre, London, ON, Canada

John D. Lubahn, MD Department of Orthopaedic Surgery, UPMC-Hamot, Erie, PA, USA

Nathan A. Monaco, MD Department of Orthopaedic Surgery, UPMC-Hamot, Erie, PA, USA

Clifford T. Pereira, MD, FRCS (Eng) Division of Plastic Surgery, Department of Orthopedics, University of California–Los Angeles, Los Angeles, CA, USA

Marco Rizzo, MD Department of Orthopedic Surgery, Division of Hand Surgery, Mayo Clinic, Rochester, MN, USA

Scott W. Rogers, MD Department of Orthopaedic Surgery, UPMC - Hamot, Erie, PA, USA

Mario Igor Rosello, MD Department of Hand Surgery, San Paolo Hospital, Savona, Italy

Vasileios I. Sakellariou, MD, MSc, PhD Department of Orthopedic Surgery, Attikon University Hospital, Athens, Greece

Anthony Smith, MD Mayo Clinic Hospital, Phoenix, AZ, USA

Panayotis N. Soucacos, MD, FACS The "Panayotis N. Soucacos" Orthopaedic Research & Education Center, Attikon University Hospital, National & Kapodistrian University of Athens, Athens, Greece

Ombretta Spingardi, MD Department of Hand Surgery, San Paolo Hospital, Savona, Italy

Peter J. Stern, MD Department of Orthopaedic Surgery, College of Medicine, University of Cincinnati, Cincinnati, OH, USA

Justin D. Stull, BA Sidney Kimmel Medical College at Thomas Jefferson University, Thomas Jefferson University Hospital, Philadelphia, PA, USA

Michael A. Tonkin, MD Department of Hand Surgery & Peripheral Nerve Surgery, Royal North Shore Hospital, University of Sydney, St. Leonards, NSW, Australia

Jeffrey Yao, MD Department of Orthopaedic Surgery, Stanford University Medical Center, Redwood City, CA, USA

Aristides B. Zoubos, MD The "Panayotis N. Soucacos" Orthopaedic Research & Education Center, Attikon University Hospital, National & Kapodistrian University of Athens, Athens, Greece

Chapter 1
Nonoperative Management of Finger Flexion Contracture in Dupuytren's Disease: Orthotic Intervention and Tissue Mobilization Techniques

Juliana Larocerie-Salgado and John S.D. Davidson

Introduction

Not all patients with deformational Dupuytren's disease are necessarily suitable candidates for surgical or medical/enzymatic management. Not only may there be contraindications due to associated medical comorbidities or the socioeconomic burdens of cost of treatment and/or time off work, but there are some disease presentations in particular that lend themselves to unpredictable and frequently unsatisfactory outcomes. Nowhere is this more evident than for disease associated with contractures of the proximal interphalangeal joints (PIPJ) of the little and ring fingers, where surgical intervention can sometimes result in recurrence or worsening of

J. Larocerie-Salgado, MSc, OT Reg (Ont)
Department of Hand Therapy, Roth-McFarlane Hand and Upper Limb Centre,
St. Joseph's Health Care Centre,
268 Grosvenor Street, London, ON, Canada, N6H 3X5
e-mail: jularocerie@hotmail.com

J.S.D. Davidson, MD, FRCSC (✉)
Division of Plastic Surgery, Hotel Dieu Hospital,
166 Brock St., Kingston, ON, Canada, K7L 5G2
e-mail: davidsoj@hdh.kari.net

© Springer International Publishing Switzerland 2016
M. Rizzo (ed.), *Dupuytren's Contracture*,
DOI 10.1007/978-3-319-23841-8_1

the contracture, decreased range of motion, dystrophic pain, and protracted rehabilitation [1–5].

At the same time, it is not as if there is nothing that can be offered to these patients. We have determined that the application of simple low load forces through the use of orthosis, stretching exercises and massage, can in most situations help stabilize the progression and in some cases improve the general state of the deformity, particularly in early presentations of the disease [6].

Case Presentation

A 71-year-old right-handed man presented to the hand clinic with a 4-year history of palpable nodules and progressive flexion contractures of the little finger bilaterally. He underwent an open fasciectomy in the left hand, with close to full correction of the flexion deformity and excellent hand function, with complete recovery after 8 weeks. To address the flexion contracture in the right little finger, he instead elected to undergo a trial of nonoperative intervention, to avoid the protracted recovery he experienced with the surgery on his other hand.

The intervention protocol comprised fabrication of an extension orthosis, to be worn at nighttime, and the demonstration of tissue mobilization techniques, including friction massage and gentle, prolonged extension stretches to be carried out over the course of the day [6]. Patients enrolled in this protocol were seen 0, 2, 4, and 6 months for review, adjustments, encouragement, and goniometry measurements of joint deformation. Ultrasound imaging, including elastography, was conducted before and after the intervention protocol in an attempt to objectively measure the dimensions and consistency of the diseased fascia [7].

Diagnosis/Assessment

Physical examination of the right hand demonstrated that the diseased fascia affected both the PIP and MCP joints of the little finger only, resulting in moderate flexion contractures of both joints (Fig. 1.1).

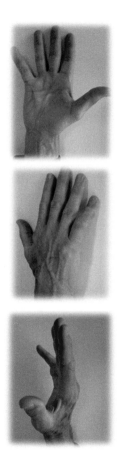

Fig. 1.1 Finger extension at the time of initial assessment

Measurements of active extension using a stainless steel finger goniometer revealed a total active extension of 50°, in which the MCP joint showed 25° of active extension, the PIP joint, 25°, and the DIP joint, 0°. In order to ensure that the flexor tendon and Dupuytren's cord were slack, MCP extension was measured with the PIP in a relaxed, slightly flexed position, and PIP joint extension with the MCP joint in flexion [8, 9].

Ultrasound imaging conducted before the initial assessment showed a long nodule over the fifth ray, distal to the distal palmar crease, measuring $28.6 \times 4.0 \times 5.6$ mm (volume = 335.4 mm^3). Ultrasound elastography was also performed providing a characterization of the consistency of the diseased fascia being measured.

Management

Following initial assessment, the patient was placed in a static hand-based volar extension orthosis, with an adjustable strap placed over involved PIP joint, as shown in Fig. 1.2. He was instructed to wear the orthosis at nighttime (6–8 h a day) subjecting the contracted tissues to prolonged application of low load forces,

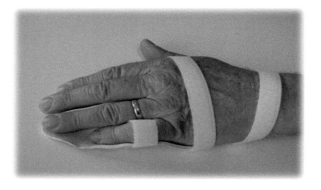

Fig. 1.2 Sample of hand-based volar extension static orthosis

while permitting unrestricted use of the hand during the day. The patient was also instructed to perform stretching exercises of the MCP and PIP joints into extension within a pain-free range and friction massage to contracted tissue (i.e., nodules and cords) throughout the course of the day.

At his 2-month visit, the orthosis was adjusted to increase extension and create a minimal space between the orthosis and the volar aspect of the PIP joint. The MCP joint was placed in as much extension as possible, and a wider strap was placed over this joint. The intent of these measures was to provide for the application of progressive low load extension forces over the involved joints during the course of therapy. Stretching and massage exercises were reviewed and emphasized.

At the time of the 4- and 6-month visit, the orthosis was further adjusted to accommodate for any improvement in extension.

Outcome

The patient had an improvement of approximately 15° in total active extension following the 6-month intervention protocol. At that time, his PIPJ extended to 15°, and the MCP joint to 20° (Table 1.1; Fig. 1.3).

Ultrasound imaging at the completion of the intervention protocol showed a reduction in the size of the nodule, which by then measured $9.7 \times 4.1 \times 5.6$ mm representing a greater than 60% decrease in measurable volume of the disease (116.6 mm^3).

Table 1.1 MCP and PIP joints extension at the time of the first and last clinic visits

	Pre-intervention	Post-intervention
MCP ext	25	20
PIP ext	25	15
DIP ext	0	0
Nodule volume	335.4 mm^3	116.6 mm^3

Post Treatment

Pre Treatment

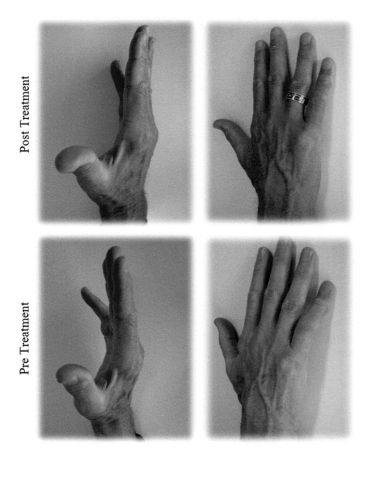

Fig. 1.3 Finger extension, pre- and post-intervention (lateral view and tabletop test)

Changes in the measurement parameters of the ultrasound elastography suggested a compositional softening of the diseased fascia over this time, as noted by decreased red coloration within the demarcated borders of the diseased fascia (Fig. 1.4).

Clinical Pearls/Pitfalls

Outcomes from surgical management of flexion contractures in Dupuytren's disease, and of the PIPJ in the little finger in particular, are at best inconsistent [1, 4]. Once considered an absolute indication for surgical intervention, PIPJ contractures are approached with surgical foreboding with suboptimal correction or stabilization of the progression of the disease often being the modest therapeutic goal [2, 8–10]. The experience at our center has been no different and consequently we have considered alternative approaches to the management of contractures particularly in the early stages of presentation. We have determined that low load force application techniques though conventional orthosis and stretching exercises in patients with mild to moderate flexion contractures, particularly of the PIPJ, can obviate or at least delay surgical intervention [6].

Our experience challenges a long held dogma that massage, stretching, and splinting are of little or no benefit in the primary management of Dupuytren's disease. It has even been argued that the application of tension load forces to Dupuytren's related contractures may in fact be counterproductive and potentially accelerate the progression of deformity [11]. However, this has always seemed counterintuitive given the demonstrated benefit of static orthosis and the application of longitudinal load forces on collagen remodeling in traumatic scars not to mention their important role in rehabilitation of patients undergoing surgical treatment of Dupuytren's. Notwithstanding our treatment protocol of nighttime orthosis and tissue mobilization, is based on an established premise of tissue remodeling shown to be related to the exposure to a maximum tolerable, prolonged low load torque applied at its end range [12, 13].

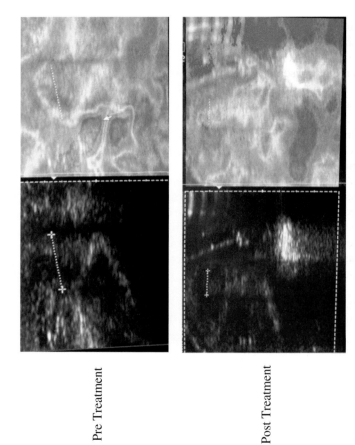

Pre Treatment

Post Treatment

Fig. 1.4 Pre- and post-treatment sagittal images of focal fibromatosis superficial to the fifth MCP joint. On the elastography images (colored), *red*=hard tissue, *blue*=soft tissue

The use of external physical forces to address contracted fascia is not an original concept in the management of Dupuytren's disease. Elliot [14] noted that as early as 1826, Charles Boyer, a "not impartial" contemporary of Dupuytren had outlined in his important *Traite des Maladies Chirurgicales* that "one can perhaps stop the progression of the disease in its early stages by placing on the dorsum of the finger a small splint fixed with a bandage, and applying lotion and relaxants to the palm of the hand."

More recently the principle of primary static stretch in Dupuytren's disease has been applied, with the aid of fairly elaborate skeletal traction devices, to people with advanced disease as a precursor to surgical correction to reduce preoperative deformity, especially at the PIPJ, stretching the skin to avert the need for skin grafting or flaps, and gradually elongate the neurovascular structures [8, 15–18]. There have also been reports of treatment of remaining flexion contractures in the PIPJ following collagenase injection with the continuous use of orthosis [19, 20].

As we have gained experience with this modality, not only have we noted improvements in the degree of joint deformity and range of motion, as demonstrated in this case presentation, we have also noted changes in the quantitative as well as qualitative nature of the disease in the fascia. Although some might argue that our observations may be due to stretching of other underlying contracted tissues, we have specifically seen, using ultrasound imaging modalities, measurable volume loss and softening of the Dupuytren's disease in many patients. In a recent series, we observed an average decrease of over 30 % in the volume of disease in the fascia (unpublished data).

Patients have frequently commented that the fascia seems softer and more compliant while undergoing treatment. Additionally, Christie and colleagues [21] demonstrated an increase in ROM and decrease in the visual appearance of fibrous adhesions associated with Dupuytren's disease with the use of cross-frictional massage. While difficult to objectively demonstrate changes in the consistency of Dupuytren's fascia, there is anatomical data from light microscopy as well as biochemical studies corroborating changes in clinical consistency of palpable disease following the application of static stretching with skeletal traction devices [8, 15–18].

Instead we have used Ultrasound Elastography to monitor changes in the mechanical consistency of the diseased fascia. It is a medical imaging modality that maps the elastic properties of soft tissue. The main premise is to distinguish whether tissue is hard or soft to give diagnostic information about the presence or status of disease. Using Elastography we have consistently observed changes in the fascia over the course of the therapy to suggest favorable changes in consistency of the disease.

As is the case for surgery, administering nonsurgical modalities also relies on careful patient selection. This relates to patient motivation and adherence, not to mention a clear understanding of the therapeutic goals of the intervention. Such is the case for prescribing a protracted rehabilitation therapy protocol involving frequent and repetitive massage and stretching of the digits and the consistent use of an orthosis to be worn at night. As well the success of the treatment would appear to depend on the extent and pattern of disease or deformity. It seems that our protocol is most effective for patients with mild to moderate degrees of contracture isolated to one or two fingers, and who simply wish to maintain their current level of function without having to submit to surgery or other medical interventions. The most consistent results in our population were seen in patients with isolated PIPJ flexion contracture that could fully adhere to the orthosis regimen. Those with more diffuse presentation of Dupuytren's disease or having difficulty adhering to the proposed treatment showed minimal or no improvement [6].

In summary, mild to moderate flexion contractures associated with Dupuytren's disease are responsive to the application of prolonged, low load forces. The use of a nighttime extension orthosis combined with intermittent stretching exercises and massage to contracted tissue can delay the progression and frequently improve the degree and consistency of flexion contractures primarily of the PIPJ. This protocol can be considered an effective alternative management strategy, at least in the short term, for those who may not want or be suitable for other types of interventions surgical or otherwise. The time course for the use of an orthosis protocol, patient selection, combination with adjuvant therapies, and management of treatment failures still remain to be determined.

Acknowledgements The authors would like to thank Dr. Paul Fenton, MD Radiologist, and Kim Fletcher, US technician, for their invaluable contribution to this project.

References

1. Denkler K. Surgical complication associated with fasciectomy for Dupuytren's disease: a 20-year review of the English literature. Eplasty. 2010;10:e15.
2. Eaton C. Evidence-based medicine: Dupuytren contracture. Plast Reconstr Surg. 2014;133:1241–51.
3. Townley WA, Baker R, Sheppard N, Grobbelaar AO. Dupuytren's unfolded. BMJ. 2006;332(7538):397–400.
4. Weinzneig N, Culver JE, Fleeger EJ. Severe contractures of the PIP joint in Dupuytren's disease: combined fasciectomy with capsuloligamentous release versus fasciectomy alone. Plast Reconstr Surg. 1996;97:560–6.
5. Worrell M. Dupuytren's disease. Orthopedics. 2012;35(1):52–60.
6. Larocerie-Salgado J, Davidson J. Nonoperative treatment of PIPJ flexion contractures associated with Dupuytren's disease. J Hand Surg Eur Vol. 2012;37(8):722–7.
7. Dewall RJ. Ultrasound elastography: principles, techniques, and clinical applications. Crit Rev Biomed Eng. 2013;41(1):1–19.
8. Engstrand C, Krevers B, Nylander G, Kvist J. Hand function and quality of life before and after fasciectomy for Dupuytren contracture. J Hand Surg Am. 2014;39(7):1333–43.
9. Hurst L. Dupuytren's contracture. In: Wolfe SW, Hotchkiss RN, Pederson WC, Kozin SH, editors. Green's operative hand surgery, vol 5, cap 5. Philadelphia: Elsevier; 2011. p. 141–58.
10. Agee JM, Goss BC. The use of skeletal extension torque in reversing Dupuytren contractures of the proximal interphalangeal joint. J Hand Surg. 2012;37A:1467–74.
11. Bisson MA, Mudera V, McGrouther DA, Grobbelaar AO. The contractile properties and responses to tensional loading of Dupuytren's disease-derived fibroblasts are altered: a cause of the contracture? Plast Reconstr Surg. 2004;113:611–21.
12. Flowers KR, LaStayo P. Effect of total end range time on improving passive range of motion. J Hand Ther. 1994;7:150–7.
13. Glasglow C, Wilton J, Tooth J. Optimal daily total end range time for contracture: resolution in hand splinting. J Hand Ther. 2003;16:207–18.
14. Elliot D. The early history of contracture of the palmar fascia: Part 1: the origin of the disease: the curse of the MacCrimmons: the hand of benediction: Cline's contracture. J Hand Surg Br. 1988;13:246–53.

15. Bailey AJ, Tarlton JF, Van der Stappen J, Sims TJ, Messina A. The continuous elongation technique for severe Dupuytren's disease. A biochemical mechanism. J Hand Surg Br. 1994;19:522–7.
16. Brandes G, Messina A, Reale E. The palmar fascia after treatment by the continuous extension technique for Dupuytren's contracture. J Hand Surg Br. 1994;19:528–33.
17. Messina A, Messina J. The continuous elongation treatment by the TEC device for severe Dupuytren's contracture of the fingers. Plast Reconstr Surg. 1993;92:84–90.
18. Rajesh KR, Rex C, Mehdi H, et al. Severe Dupuytren's contracture of the proximal interphalangeal joint: treatment by two-stage technique. J Hand Surg Br. 2000;25(B):442–4.
19. Skirven TM, Bachoura A, Jacoby SM, et al. The effect of a therapy protocol for increasing correction of severely contracted proximal interphalangeal joints caused by Dupuytren Disease and treated with collagenase injection. J Hand Surg. 2013;38A:684–9.
20. Sweet S, Blackmore S. Surgical and therapy update on the management of Dupuytren's disease. J Hand Ther. 2014;27:77–84.
21. Christie WS, Puhl AA, Lucaciu OC. Cross-frictional therapy and stretching for the treatment of palmar adhesions due to Dupuytren's contracture: a prospective study. Man Ther. 2012;17:479–82.

Chapter 2
Needle Aponeurotomy in the Management of Dupuytren's Contracture

Clifford T. Pereira and Prosper Benhaim

Introduction

Dupuytren's contractures (DC) is a benign fibroproliferative disorder of the fascia of the hand and fingers, resulting in progressive thickening and shortening of the palmar fascia. This results in the formation of cords, flexion deformities of the digits, and ultimately loss of range of motion, especially loss of functional finger extension [1]. The aim of surgical intervention involves the preservation and improvement of hand function by either division of (fasciotomy) or removal of (fasciectomy) the diseased tissue. Standard treatment

C.T. Pereira, MD, FRCS (Eng) • P. Benhaim, MD (✉)
Department of Orthopedics Surgery and Division of Plastic Surgery,
University of California–Los Angeles, Box 957326,
10945 LeConte Avenue, Room 33-55 PVUB,
Los Angeles, CA 90095-7326, USA
e-mail: cpereira72@yahoo.com; pbenhaim@mednet.ucla.edu

© Springer International Publishing Switzerland 2016   13
M. Rizzo (ed.), *Dupuytren's Contracture*,
DOI 10.1007/978-3-319-23841-8_2

indications include metacarpophalangeal (MCP) joint contracture
of greater than 30° and/or any proximal interphalangeal (PIP) joint
contracture. Current treatment options for DC include open fasciectomy (OF), limited fasciectomy (LF), needle aponeurotomy
(NA), and Clostridial collagenase injections. Percutaneous needle
fasciotomy or needle aponeurotomy (NA) is a minimally invasive
technique that uses a small hypodermic needle as a percutaneous
scalpel blade to perforate, weaken, and/or divide the cord to the
point where finger manipulation can result in rupture of the cord
and improvement in finger extension. This chapter focuses on the
use of NA, its indications, advantages, disadvantages, technical
pearls, and literature review. A detailed discussion on other treatment options including open fasciectomy or collagenase injections
is beyond the scope of this chapter and will be presented in other
chapters. Pertinent comparisons between NA and other treatment
options, however, will be discussed.

Case Presentation

History

The patient is a 72-year-old right hand dominant retired aerospace
engineer who presented with a 10-year history of bilateral hand
Dupuytren's contractures. The right side was worse than the left,
with progressive worsening of the contractures over the previous
year. The contractures had advanced to a point where they interfered with his ability to play tennis and a number of other activities
of daily living. The patient had had no prior treatment for this on
either hand. He had no numbness or tingling. He did not remember
any specific inciting event or trauma. His family history was nega-
tive for DC. His ancestry included French and Belgian lineage. He
denied any involvement of the soles of his feet (Ledderhose disease) or shaft of his penis (Peyronie's disease). He was not diabetic
or epileptic. He denied abuse of tobacco or recreational drugs, and
consumed alcohol only socially.

Examination

The *right* hand had evidence of Dupuytren's disease, including a distal first web space commissural cord and pretendinous cords over the first, second, third, fourth, and fifth metacarpals. The most predominant of these was the fifth metacarpal pretendinous cord. There was no natatory cord formation in the web spaces. The right thumb had a radial lateral cord at the radial border of the proximal phalanx, with a Dupuytren's nodule at the A1 pulley level. The ring finger had an ulnar lateral cord at the ulnar border of the proximal phalanx. The small finger had a radial lateral cord at the radial border of the proximal/middle phalanges and a central cord at the proximal/middle phalanx level. The small finger also had a Dupuytren's nodule at the A1 pulley level and at the proximal phalanx level. There were no dorsal proximal interphalangeal joint Garrod's pads noted. Contractures in the right hand included 15° at the middle finger MP joint, 35° at the ring finger MP joint, 85° at the small finger MP joint, 60° at the small finger PIP joint, and 30° at the small finger DIP joint. The other finger joints of the right hand had full extension and all joints had full flexion. Sensation was intact in all digits. No triggering of any of the digits was noted. All extensor and flexor tendons were intact, without any evidence for extensor tendon subluxation or sagittal band rupture (Fig. 2.1).

The *left* hand had evidence of Dupuytren's disease, including a distal first web space contracture cord and pretendinous cords over the first, second, third, fourth, and fifth metacarpals. The fifth metacarpal pretendinous cord was the most prominent cord. There was no natatory cord formation in the web spaces. The small finger had a central cord at the proximal phalanx level and nodule formation over the A1 pulley and proximal phalanx in the small finger. There were no Garrod's pads noted. Contractures in the left hand included 15° at the ring finger MP joint and 50° at the small finger MP joint. The other finger joints of the left hand had full extension and all joints had full flexion. Sensation was intact in all digits. No triggering of any of the digits was noted. All extensor and flexor tendons were intact, without any evidence for extensor tendon subluxation or sagittal band rupture.

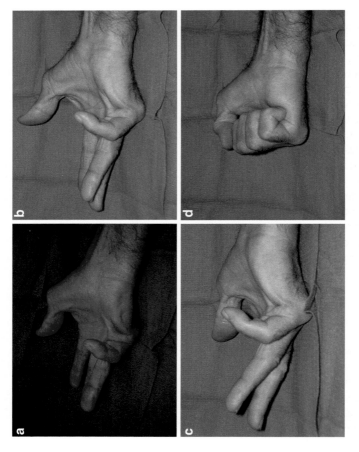

Fig. 2.1 Dupuytren's contracture of *right* hand—before needle aponeurotomy. (**a**) anterior-posterior view, (**b**) oblique view, (**c**) lateral view, (**d**) composite fist

Diagnosis and Assessment

The patient had bilateral hand Dupuytren's disease involving both MP and PIP joints, right side worse than left. Treatment options offered to the patient included conservative management with splints and hand therapy vs. needle aponeurotomy vs. a combination of needle aponeurotomy and limited fasciectomy vs. open palmar fasciectomy vs. collagenase injection. The relative advantages, disadvantages, potential complications, and alternatives of each of these approaches were discussed with the patient in detail. The patient carefully considered these options and elected to undergo needle aponeurotomy (NA). Specific to NA, in addition to general procedure-related risks, the patient was explained that it is a blind percutaneous procedure that carries a risk of injury to nerves, vessels, tendons, and a higher risk of recurrence when compared to conventional Dupuytren's contracture release surgery. We also explained the risk of skin tears that may occur as a result of the procedure, which would necessitate local wound care postoperatively. Such skin tears can take 1–4 weeks to heal fully, depending on their size and location. Finally, the patient also understood that no surgical approach, whether conventional or needle aponeurotomy, could guarantee full range of motion following surgery, either immediately or in the long run.

Management and Outcome

The patient underwent NA initially on the *right* hand (Fig. 2.2). The fifth metacarpal pretendinous cord was approached first at the proximal portion of the palm and extended all the way to the MP flexion crease of the small finger. Caution was taken to remain central on the cord in order to avoid injury to the nearby neurovascular bundles. In addition, care was taken to avoid going too deeply with the needle in order to avoid injury to the underlying flexor tendons and neurovascular structures. With each pass of the needle, there was progressive release of the Dupuytren's contracture in the small finger, especially at the MP joint. A nearly identical procedure was repeated for the second, third, and fourth metacarpal

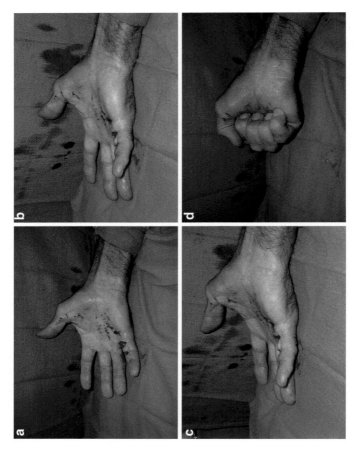

Fig. 2.2 Dupuytren's contracture of *right* hand—immediately after needle aponeurotomy, (**a**) anterior-posterior view, (**b**) lateral view, (**c**) composite fist

pretendinous cords, as well as for the first metacarpal pretendinous cord extending to the thumb. The first web space contracture cords were also released in this fashion. The Dupuytren's contracture in the small finger was next addressed at the proximal and middle phalanx level using the same needle aponeurotomy technique, this time addressing the central cord and radial lateral cord at the proximal and middle phalanx level. As in the palm, great care was taken to avoid injury to the neurovascular structures and to the underlying flexor tendons. Marked improvement was achieved in extension of both the PIP and DIP joints with this technique. In a similar fashion, the ring finger Dupuytren's contracture release was performed at the proximal phalanx level by releasing the ulnar lateral cord in the ring finger at the proximal phalanx level, at multiple locations. The right thumb radial lateral cord at the radial border of the proximal phalanx was released in a similar fashion at the thumb level, with care being taken to avoid injury to the radial digital nerve and artery. The needle aponeurotomy technique was able to achieve full extension in the thumb, index finger, middle finger, and ring finger. However, the small finger PIP joint still had a residual contracture secondary to an independent PIP joint volar capsular contracture. This was addressed at the end of the procedure, by infiltrating all the fingers with 0.5 % Marcaine to achieve a digital block in all digits. The fingers were manipulated with forceful extension to achieve completion rupture of the cords, thereby further improving extension and even hyperextension of the MP joints. In addition, we specifically performed a PIP joint closed capsulotomy to increase the extension of the small finger PIP joint. This was successful in achieving full extension of the PIP joint in the small finger. The procedure did produce several skin tears, including a skin tear at the distal palmar crease over the fifth metacarpal, a skin tear at the MP flexion crease of the small finger, and a skin tear at the PIP flexion crease of the small finger. All three tears were less than 1 cm in diameter and did not involve exposure of the flexor tendon sheath or neurovascular bundles. The remaining discontinuous segments of the pretendinous cords and associated nodules were locally infiltrated with a total of 50 mg of triamcinolone to minimize the risk of a flare reaction postoperatively and to minimize the risk of recurrence. The skin tears were dressed with antibiotic ointment and a sterile soft dressing. The patient commenced supervised hand therapy on postoperative day 1, including use of a nighttime extension splint to maintain the fingers at full extension at night for 4 months following the procedure. At his 2-month postoperative visit, the patient's right hand wounds had fully healed with no residual open wounds. All extensor and flexor tendons were intact. Light touch sensation was normal in all digits. All fingers of the right hand had full range of motion, *including full active and passive extension of the digits* (Fig. 2.3). The patient subsequently returned in 5 months and had NA performed on his left hand, which was also successfully corrected. At his 2-year follow-up, his right hand still had full flexion and extension with no signs of recurrence (Fig. 2.4).

Technique

Preoperative preparation: Needle aponeurotomy can be performed in either an office setting or an outpatient surgery center, the choice of which may be dictated by patient preference, surgeon preference, and/or insurance coverage eligibility issues. Some insurance companies will require that this type of procedure be performed in a Medicare-approved procedure room, which may or may not be available in every surgeon's office. Some surgeons prefer the formal setting of an outpatient surgery center with better lighting and monitoring by a nurse. The procedure is performed under local anesthesia, without intravenous sedation, regional block, or monitored anesthesia care. Patients are asked to stop anticoagulation before the procedure, if possible. However, anticoagulation is not considered an absolute contraindication to the procedure. The patient is placed recumbent to minimize possible vasovagal responses. The technique is explained to the patient in detail, including the importance of reporting paresthesias that may develop during the procedure and of avoiding sudden movements. Short excursion fingertip flexion/extension is explained to the patient and demonstrated.

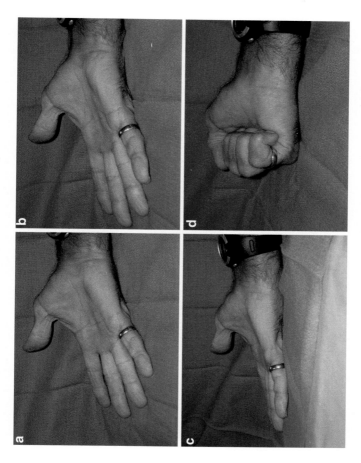

Fig. 2.3 Dupuytren's contracture of *right* hand—2 months after needle aponeurotomy, (**a**) anterior-posterior view, (**b**) oblique view, (**c**) lateral *view*, (**d**) composite fist

C.T. Pereira and P. Benhaim

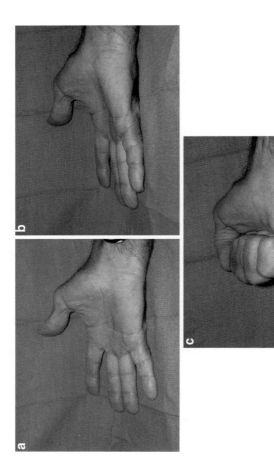

Fig. 2.4 Dupuytren's contracture of *right* hand—2 years after needle aponeurotomy, (**a**) anterior-posterior view, (**b**) lateral view, (**c**) composite fist

Local anesthetic field block: Sensory end organs of the skin are located in the deep dermis, but the subdermal fat, palmar aponeurosis, and cords are insensate. Digital nerves are sensitive to pressure or direct contact; joint capsules and flexor tendon sheaths are innervated as well [2]. Thus, vital structures are sensate and cords are not, allowing NA to be performed safely under local anesthesia. This also makes it imperative that just the skin overlying the cords is blocked by the local anesthetic injected, performing a superficial intradermal anesthetic injection only and carefully avoiding deeper injection that may block the digital nerves. It is critical that the subcutaneous tissues and underlying nerves are not blocked, since that would eliminate the ability of the nerves to respond to direct contact. As the NA procedure is performed, since it is a blind procedure that does not allow direct visualization of the digital nerves, the primary method by which one avoids injury to the underlying nerves is to rely on a Tinel's type of response from the nerve if the needle comes into contact or even just close proximity to the nerve. Report by the fully awake patient of Tinel's-like paresthesias would indicate that the needle is too close to the nerve, allowing the surgeon to redirect the needle to another location and avoid injury to the digital nerves. This is especially important in high-risk areas such as spiral cords at the base of fingers, where digital nerves can be displaced from their normal anatomical location.

To achieve the local dermal block, the upper extremity is prepped and draped in the usual sterile fashion. Under standard sterile and antiseptic conditions, the selected area is infiltrated with 1 % lidocaine (with 1:100,000 epinephrine) in a 3 ml syringe with a luer lock and a short 30-gauge needle in order to achieve the local dermal block. Infiltration pain can be reduced by buffering the local anesthetic with sodium bicarbonate. For precise surface anesthesia, 0.05–0.1 ml intradermal injections are infiltrated at multiple focal positions along the entire length of the cords targeted for release (Fig. 2.5). Despite careful technique, anesthetic diffusion can cause partial digital nerve block. Loss of light touch denoting complete digital nerve block may be an indication that the procedure may need to be aborted until such time that light touch returns. To minimize this possibility, some surgeons will advocate a progressive sequential local anesthetic injection approach, starting distally, releasing a portion of the cords distally, and then subsequent more

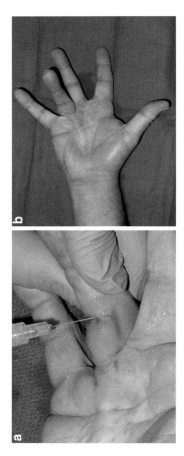

Fig. 2.5 (**a**) Local anesthetic injection technique demonstrating intradermal injection. (**b**) Blanched skin demonstrating area injected with 1 % lidocaine with 1:100,000 epinephrine

proximal local anesthetic injection in multiple stages. With this modification, the Tinel's sign response proximally can be preserved, even if the distal portion of the nerve is inadvertently blocked. No tourniquet is required for the procedure.

Technique: The needle aponeurotomy is performed with a hypodermic needle, with different surgeons preferring different gauged needles ranging in size from 25-gauge to 18 gauge. The smaller-25 gauge needle will typically be employed using a combination of perforation and sweeping maneuvers designed to weaken the cords, while a larger 18-gauge needle is more typically utilized as a percutaneous fasciotome in a windshield wiper back and forth fashion with the goal to create a transverse percutaneous fasciotomy. Treatment portals are best planned in areas of maximal bowstringing of cords, especially if the cords become more taut on joint extension [3]. Nodules are firm regardless of joint position and should be avoided unless directly contributing to the contracture and only if proven to be so after proximal and/or distal non-nodular cord segments are released [3]. Placing portals over flexor creases is not preferred due to the proximity of the flexor sheath and the increased likelihood of skin tears, although release at creases is sometimes necessary for successful release. Cords are tensioned, palpated, and pinched between the fingertips of the surgeon's non-dominant hand to stabilize the cord. Gentle skin traction is placed over the cords to accentuate the bowstringing of the cord, thus pulling the cord away from deeper structures. Extreme extension of the finger is avoided and the patient asked to relax the fingers to keep the flexor tendons slack, reducing the risk of inadvertent tendon injury. This is especially important at the volar aspect of the MP joint, where hyperextension of the MP joint brings the flexor tendons in close approximation to the overlying skin in the region of the distal palmar crease, placing the flexor tendons at greater risk for injury or even complete transection [3].

Fasciotomy portals are usually made equal to the cord width. Once the dermis is penetrated, the needle is oriented tangentially to create a plane between the dermis and cord. The needle tip is then reoriented perpendicular to the cord's longitudinal axis, with the bevel transverse to the cord. A repeated side-to-side sweeping movement is made with the needle tip to graze or scratch the cord.

If using a smaller 25-gauge needle, multiple perforations of the cord are also used to weaken the cord for subsequent manipulation/ cord rupture at the end of the procedure. A constant proprioceptive feedback is obtained during the cord division. This is in the form of a gristly and firm feel with a concomitant scraping sound as the needle scratches through the cord. The needle is changed frequently to maintain sharpness. The end point of the fasciotomy at each point is reached when firm feedback at the needle tip stops, and further gentle probing yields a soft feel. A "trampoline" fingertip bouncing can also be used to assess the adequacy of the cord rupture [3].

Some surgeons prefer release that commences proximally and progresses distally to the MP and/or PIP joints, as required. Others prefer a distal-to-proximal technique. Portals are placed an average of 5 mm apart. Care is taken to remain central on the cord in order to avoid injury to the adjacent neurovascular bundles. Care is also taken to avoid going too deeply in order to avoid injury to the underlying flexor tendons and neurovascular structures, including superficial palmar arch and proximal branches of the median and/ or ulnar nerves as they exit from the carpal and ulnar tunnels, respectively. Fingertip sensation to light touch stimulation is repeatedly checked throughout the procedure. Each pass with the needle is made deliberately, allowing the patient enough time to react. The slicing or perforating motion of the needle is stopped and the needle redirected immediately if the patient reports electric current sensation or the equivalent of a Tinel's sign down the treated finger. Tendon proximity is checked regularly by leaving the needle in place and watching for the presence or absence of needle motion with short gentle active tendon excursion.

Areas of pitting are best avoided, since portal placement can transect a dimple sinus, with higher risk for multiple skin tears in close proximity. The skin at the depths of the pits is also likely not well anesthetized, causing pain. Spiral cords usually occur at the junction of the palm and the base of the finger; caution must be exercised in these areas since they can displace the neurovascular bundle superficially and centrally. Since the neurovascular bundles are embedded in subcutaneous fat, the presence of fat between the dermis and the cord should alert the surgeon to a displaced neurovascular bundle. These areas should be avoided, if possible. Eaton describes the use of Doppler or ultrasound, especially in areas of a suspected spiral cord, to identify the neurovascular bundle [3]. The senior author does not generally use this in his practice, relying instead on Tinel's sign feedback. Finally, sometimes release of a radial or ulnar lateral cord does not result in full extension of the proximal interphalangeal joint (PIPJ). This may be secondary to a nonpalpable central extension of the cord. An additional release centrally, just proximal to the PIPJ flexion crease, usually completes the correction, although release in this area can carry higher risk for tendon injury since the central cord will often blend into the A3 pulley in this area. Some patients will also have independent PIP joint volar capsular contractures or relative shortening/tightening of the flexor tendon sheath specifically at the A3 pulley level, which may need to be addressed separately during the manipulation portion of the procedure.

Final manipulation: Once the cords have been adequately weakened/divided at multiple sites, the patient is tested in a formal fashion to confirm that all flexor tendons (individual testing of the flexor digitorum superficialis and profundus tendons going to each digit) and all individual digital nerves remain intact. Once so verified, the treated sites are injected with local anesthetic to achieve combined palmar and digital blocks that will allow forceful manipulation of the fingers without significant pain. Our preference is to use 0.5 % bupivacaine without epinephrine, while others prefer 1 % lidocaine instead. After good digital block and palmar anesthesia has been established, the fingers are passively stretched to achieve completion rupture of the cords and to break any residual tethering. The wrist should be flexed as the finger is being extended to minimize risk of tendon rupture [3]. Manipulation of the digits under local anesthesia also allows release of a tight flexor tendon sheath and/or PIP joint closed volar capsulotomy, as needed. Intra-articular local anesthetic injection of the PIP and MCP joints has been employed by some prior to the final manipulation, after all needle manipulations are completed. This enables the patient to tolerate a greater amount of force during the finger extension process to facilitate residual cord rupture, and enhance the results.

Post-procedure: Once all cords have been released, nodules and segmental areas of the released cords can be injected with depot corticosteroid such as triamcinolone acetate 10 mg/cc or beta-methasone 6 mg/cc to minimize the risk of recurrence and to minimize the risk of a Dupuytren's flare reaction postoperatively. Skin tears are dressed with ample antibiotic ointment to prevent desiccation of underlying structures, nonadherent gauze (e.g., Xeroform gauze), and a light gauze bandage. Coverage with antibiotic ointment to prevent tissue desiccation is especially critical if there is any exposed tendon noted at the base of a skin tear. The patient is instructed to change the dressings after 48 h, and daily thereafter. Depending on the severity of the initial contracture, the hand may be placed in a volar short arm splint extending to the finger tips, with the involved digits placed at full extension. The patient is referred to hand therapy for active flexion and extension range of motion exercises and gentle passive extension stretching. Heavy grasping is deferred until the wounds have healed completely. Nighttime extension splinting is continued for 6–16 weeks.

Literature Review

Dupuytren's contracture was first described by a Swiss physician—Felix Plater, in his book titled "Observationum in Hominis Affectibus" in 1614. Sir Henry Cline, in 1777, recognized the involvement of the palmar fascia and described the first treatment of this disease, which consisted of division of the pathologic cords, although he incorrectly conceptualized the underlying cause of the palmar fascia contracture as secondary to trauma to the underlying tendons [4]. Later in 1831, a French military surgeon—Baron Guillaume Dupuytren—described and operated on the palmar fibrosis that now takes his name [5]. The first closed percutaneous fasciotomy was performed by Cooper in 1822. The technique now bears his name—Coopers fasciotomy [3]. With the advent of anesthesia, Goyrand [6] introduced limited fasciectomy (LF); and Fergusson [7] introduced open fasciectomy (OF). Thereafter, surgery became more aggressive until the 1950s, when total palmar fasciectomy was popularized by McIndoe and Beare [8]. However, the high complication rates associated with this technique forced surgeons to return to LFs. J. Vernon Luck reestablished the concept of a percutaneous fasciotomy approach in 1959 with a specially designed percutaneous fasciotome (Luck fasciotome). It was not until 1972, however, that French rheumatologists Lermusiaux and Debeyre [9] reintroduced and repopularized the Cooper fasciotomy, but performed it using 25-gauge needles under local anesthesia. They called it *percutaneous needle fasciotomy* (PNF). The technique is now also called Needle Aponeurotomy (NA).

Currently, the four requirements to perform NA in Dupuytren's disease as described by Eaton [3] include (1) a contracture, secondary to a (2) palpable cord that lies beneath (3) redundant skin, in a (4) cooperative patient. It should not be performed in the absence of a palpable cord or overlying scarred tissue/skin, although prior surgery or scar tissue is not an absolute contraindication if there is still an appropriate and identifiable cord that can be safely released by NA. Needle aponeurotomy should not be performed on contractures not due to Dupuytren's disease, such as postsurgical scarring, PIP joint volar capsular contractures, scleroderma-related contracture, or burn scar contractures. It should also be performed with particular precaution in PIP joint contractures when there is a large nodule or cord between the PIPJ flexion crease and the proximal digital crease [10]. Finally, NA should never be performed in infiltrative disease, Dupuytren's diathesis, or constitutionally treatment-resistant Dupuytren's, since this will likely result in rapid recurrence [11]. Young age is a relative contraindication for NA, due to the high likelihood of recurrence and a relatively more aggressive disease presentation in the patient who presents at a younger age.

Several groups of surgeons and rheumatologists have reported the French experience with NA [12–15]. In 1993, Badois et al. performed NA in 138 patients and found that 81 % had good or excellent primary results with a Tubiana Class I or II Dupuytren's contracture. In the group of patients with Tubiana stage IV disease, 48 % had good results. There were no major complications, although there was skin tear in 16 %, digital dysesthesia in 2 %, and infection in 2 % [12]. Bleton et al. documented the results of a prospective study of NA on 59 patients [13]. Sixty-one percent of patients had a good result, with an improvement of more than 50 %. Lermusiaux et al. reported the results of a large experience with NA, with an improvement of over 70 % in 81 % of hands. The complication rate was 0.05 % for both tendon and digital nerve injuries [14]. Foucher et al. reported an average 79 % gain in extension for the MCP joints and 65 % for the PIP joints in their cohort of patients. All complications were minor, including skin tear in 4 %, temporary paresthesias in 2 %, and superficial infection in 1 % [15].

It should be noted that published studies on Dupuytren's contracture tend to use a variety of definitions of both correction of contracture and recurrence [10–18]. For instance, Hueston's definition for Dupuytren's contracture recurrence was the most widely accepted definition. Hueston used "appearance of new Dupuytren's tissue within the area cleared at operation" [19]. This definition, however, could not be utilized in NA treatment series, since tissue is never removed. This makes it difficult to compare the results of NA with other techniques. Older studies therefore never clearly defined recurrence in Dupuytren's disease [12–15]. Van Rijssen et al. redefined recurrence indirectly, as an increase of the total passive extension deficit of 30° or more in a ray [16]. A worsening of digital extension of 30° was chosen because it corresponds to the Hueston tabletop test and is considered the minimal contracture required to qualify for surgery. This measure is reproducible and clinically more relevant. The issue of recurrence of disease versus progression of disease in previously untreated areas of the hand is not necessarily well defined in the literature, as well.

Needle aponeurotomy has also been tried in recurrent Dupuytren's disease. Van Rijssen et al. performed a retrospective review of recurrent Dupuytren's disease (defined as total passive extension deficit (TPED) of at least 30° in one or more rays) in patients previously treated with NA or LF. Needle aponeurotomy was performed on all these patients. They found NA to be especially effective for the MCP joint, with an average improvement in TPED of 93 % at MP joints, compared to 57 % in PIP joints. They concluded that NA leads to good immediate results for both post-NA and post-LF recurrence. A secondary recurrence occurred in 50 % cases after 4.4 years on an average, and these were successfully treated with LF. By using NA at the first recurrence, they were able to postpone the LF procedure by 2.9 years, and the LF was not more complicated than in cases of primary disease [20].

Needle aponeurotomy has several advantages over LF and OF, namely being able to be done in an office/ambulatory surgical setting; optimal return of hand function usually within a week post-procedure; and allows both hands to be treated fairly quickly and more safely in high-risk patients (e.g., those on anticoagulants or with significant medical comorbidities that increase risk of anesthesia) [3, 10]. Disadvantages of NA include more rapid and higher overall recurrence rate than with open surgery [10]. There is also an inability to correct skin shortage and to address severe or fixed capsular contractures of the PIP joint [10]. The NA technique itself does require good knowledge of the pathologic anatomy seen in Dupuytren's contracture, with a definite learning curve associated with its adoption and application by the treating surgeon, especially in the context of a blind procedure that places digital neurovascular structures at significant risk if the technique is not performed in a precise and cautious manner.

One of the few available randomized, controlled studies showed NA and LF to be similarly effective for contracture release in lower Tubiana stages (see Table 2.1) [16]. This report also demonstrated recovery after NA to be much faster than after LF. Compared to NA, limited fasciectomy has a cumulative complication rate of 19 % [17]. Another disadvantage of LF is the relatively long recovery period of 21–58 days [18]. Despite these differences, many patients prefer NA over LF because it is minimally invasive and has a short recovery period [16].

Table 2.1 Tubiana classification of Dupuytren's contracture of the fingers

Tubiana class	TPED (°)
I	0–45
II	46–90
III	91–135
IV	>135

TPED total passive extension deficit

In 2010, the U.S. Food and Drug Administration granted American approval for clinical use of injectable collagenase produced by the *Clostridium histolyticum* species. To date, clinical efficacy and safety of Dupuytren's treatment with collagenase has been demonstrated in two double-blind, placebo-controlled studies, the Collagenase Option for Reduction of Dupuytren's I and II trials [21, 22]. The CORD I study obtained clinical success in 130 of 203 patients (64 %), with a mean of 1.7 injections required per affected joint to reach the desired end point of joint motion to within 0–5° of full extension [21]. A mean of 1.5 injections was required to achieve clinical success in 20 of 45 patients (44 %) in the CORD II study [22]. In a recent v review comparing NA to collagenase, Nydick et al. showed that short-term (3 months) clinical outcomes and patient satisfaction were equal. Both clinical success (defined as reduction of contracture to within 0–5° of normal) and mean reduction in contracture were similar between groups [23]. The number of required or recommended collagenase injections is not known and is currently being investigated. The optimum timing of post-injection manipulation after collagenase injection remains unanswered, although a number of treating physicians have manipulated the treated fingers as long as 1–2 weeks after the initial collagenase injection. Although NA can be accomplished during one office visit, as opposed to two office visits for the collagenase-treated patient, NA routinely requires more treatment time when compared with collagenase injection.

The three currently available techniques for treating Dupuytren's contracture, i.e., FA, NA, and collagenase, have been compared with regard to cost-effectiveness. Using a cost-effective treatment based on the traditional willingness-to-pay of $50,000 per quality-adjusted life years (QALY) gained, Chen et al. showed that open partial fasciectomy is not cost-effective ($820,114 per QALY gained over no treatment). Needle aponeurotomy is only cost-effective if the success rate is 100 % ($49,631 per QALY gained over no treatment). Collagenase injection is cost-effective when priced under $945 per injection ($49,995 per QALY gained over no treatment). However, if priced at market price of approximately $5400 per injection, the cost was $166,268 per QALY gained [24].

Finally, since during the initial NA, the cord is directly accessible, studies have been conducted to inject substances at the time in order to augment the outcome of NA. Depot steroid injections such as triamcinolone acetonide (TA) and autologous fat transfers have shown promising results. To answer the question if steroid injections are beneficial at the time of NA, McMillan and Binhammer performed a randomized controlled study on 47 patients with DC. Patients were randomized to either receive TA injections immediately following, 6 weeks, and 3 months after the procedure, or not receive any injections. Injections were administered into the cords. Total active extension deficit (TAED) was measured at 6 months post-procedure. There was a statistically significant improvement in TAED in the steroid-injected group (87 %), vs. the non-injected group (64 %). They conclude that at least in the short term (6 months), steroid injections improve NA outcomes. The authors also report subjective observation of fat survival, which is both palpable and visible between the skin and the released cords. They theorize that fat grafts help to decrease adhesions and separate strands of cord scar in the hand. The study did have some limitations. The short follow-up period of 6 months is not adequate to judge the long-term effectiveness of their technique. Furthermore, the baseline TAED was 103° in the steroid-injected group vs. 80° in the non-injected group. The result of increase in percentage of correction could well have been due to the greater potential for correction in the steroid-injected group. Although steroid injection may prove to be a promising adjunct to NA, longer-term studies with equivalent cohorts are therefore needed [25].

Hovius et al. reported their experience of 91 patients (99 hands) where a novel combination of percutaneous release with percutaneous autologous fat grafting was performed. The procedure consists of an extensive percutaneous aponeurotomy that completely disintegrates the cord and separates it from the dermis. Subsequently, the authors injected the subcutaneous plane of dissection with autologous lipoaspirate obtained by liposuction. Patients were placed in an extension splint for 1 week and continued with nighttime splinting for 3–6 months. The average contracture at the proximal interphalangeal joint improved significantly from 61° to 27°, and contracture at the MCP joint improved from 37° to −5°. Ninety-four percent of patients returned to normal use of the hand within 2–4 weeks and 95 % were very satisfied with the result. No new scars were added, and a supple palmar fat pad was mostly restored [26]. Thus, preliminary results appear to support autologous fat and steroid injections to augment NA outcomes. It seems likely that combinations of surgery, needle aponeurotomy, collagenase, steroids, and fat grafting will be the future of treatment for Dupuytren's contracture. Much work needs to be still done to clarify the best indications and combinations of these treatment modalities.

Clinical Pearls/Pitfalls

1. Precision superficial infiltration of local anesthetic limited to just the skin overlying the cords and not deeper structures, in order to prevent digital nerve block.
2. Abort the procedure if light touch is lost due to local anesthetic diffusion and inadvertent digital nerve block.
3. Use an appropriate needle size, based on surgeon preference, ranging from 25 gauge to 18 gauge needle.
4. Needle tip is placed perpendicular to the cord's longitudinal axis, with the bevel transverse to the cord.
5. Change needle frequently to maintain sharpness.
6. A windshield wiper back and forth slicing motion used for larger gauge needles; perforating technique for smaller gauge needles.
7. Fasciotomy portals placed at areas of maximal bowstringing of the contracture cords.
8. Avoid flexor creases or pits.
9. Avoid forceful hyperextension of fingers to tense cords, especially when releasing at the MP joint (distal palmar crease) level.
10. Monitor constantly for proprioceptive feedback.
11. Stop if patient complains of paraesthesias or resistance to the needle tip stops.
12. Release is commenced either proximally and progressing distally to the MP and/or PIP joints, or vice versa, based on surgeon preference.

13. Portals are placed an average of 5 mm apart.
14. Care is taken to remain central on the cord.
15. Fingertip sensitivity is checked repeatedly.
16. Each move is made deliberately, allowing the patient enough time to react with a possible Tinel's sign type of response that would indicate close proximity to the nerve.
17. Tendon proximity is checked regularly with short gentle active tendon excursion.
18. Once the cord has been adequately weakened/divided at multiple sites, the finger is passively stretched under local anesthesia to achieve completion rupture of the cords.
19. After final manipulation, nodules can be injected with depot corticosteroid.
20. Skin tears are dressed with ample antibiotic ointment.
21. Aggressive active/passive range of motion exercises with or without supervised hand therapy commenced as soon as possible.
22. Nighttime extension splinting continued for 6–16 weeks.

References

1. Shih B, Bayat A. Scientific understanding and clinical management of Dupuytren disease. Nat Rev Rheumatol. 2010;6:715–26.
2. Schultz RJ, Krishnamurthy S, Johnston AD. A gross anatomic and histologic study of the innervation of the proximal interphalangeal joint. J Hand Surg. 1984;9A:669–74.
3. Eaton C. Percutaneous fasciotomy for Dupuytren's contracture. J Hand Surg. 2011;36A:910–5.
4. Cline H. Notes on pathology. London: St. Thomas's Hospital Medical School Library; 1777. p. 185.
5. Elliot D. The early history of contracture of the palmar fascia. J Hand Surg. 1988;13B:246–53.
6. Goyrand G. Nouvellesrecherchessur la retraction permanente des doigts. Gazette Medicale Paris. 1883;3:481–6.
7. Fergusson W. A system of practical surgery. London: Churchill; 1842.
8. McIndoe AH, Beare RL. The surgical management of Dupuytren's contracture. Am J Surg. 1958;95:197–203.
9. Lermusiaux JL, Debeyre N. Le traitement medical de la malidie de Dupuytren. Rhumatologique. Paris: Expansion Scientifique; 1979. p. 338–43.

10. Van Rijssen AL, Gerbrandy FSJ, Linden HT, Klip H, Werker PMN. A comparison of the direct outcomes of percutaneous needle fasciotomy and limited fasciectomy for Dupuytren's disease: a 6-week follow-up study. J Hand Surg. 2006;31A:717–25.
11. Degreeef I, De Smet L. Risk factors in Dupuytren's diathesis: is recurrence after surgery predictable? In: Degreef I, editor. Therapy resisting Dupuytren's disease. New perspectives in adjuvant treatment. Leuven: KatholickeUniversiteit; 2009. p. 50–5.
12. Badois FJ, Lermusiaux C, Masse C, Kuntz D. Nonsurgical treatment of Dupuytren disease using needle fasciotomy. Rev Rhum Engl Ed. 1993; 60:692–7.
13. Bleton R, Marcireau D, Almot J-Y. Treatment of Dupuytren disease by percutaneous needle fasciotomy. In: Saffer P, Amadio PC, Foucher G, editors. Current practice in hand surgery. London: Martin Dunitz; 1997. p. 187–93.
14. Lermusiaux JL, Lellouche H, Badois F, Kuntz D. How should Dupuytren contracture be managed in 1997? Rev Rhum Engl Ed. 1997;64:775–6.
15. Foucher G, Medina J, Navarro R. Percutaneous needle aponeurotomy: complications and results. J Hand Surg. 2003;28B:427–31.
16. Van Rijssen AL, Ter Linden H, Werker PM. 5-year results of randomized clinical trial on treatment in Dupuytren's disease: percutaneous needle fasciotomy versus limited fasciectomy. Plast Reconstr Surg. 2012; 129:469–77.
17. McFarlane RM, McGrouther DA. Complications and their management. In: McFarlane RM, McGrouther DA, Flint M, editors. Dupuytren's disease: biology and treatment. Edinburgh: Churchill Livingstone; 1990. p. 377–82.
18. Rodrigo JJ, Niebauer JJ, Brown JL, Doyle JR. Treatment of Dupuytren's contracture. Long-term results after fasciotomy and fascial excision. J Bone Joint Surg. 1976;58A:380–7.
19. Hueston JT. Current state of treatment of Dupuytren's disease. Ann Chir Main. 1984;3:81–92.
20. Van Rijssen AL, Paul MN, Werker MN. Percutaneous needle fasciotomy for recurrent Dupuytren disease. J Hand Surg. 2002;37A:1820–3.
21. Hurst LC, Badalamente MA, Hentz VR, et al. Injectable collagenase clostridium histolyticum for Dupuytren's contracture. N Engl J Med. 2009;361(3):968–79.
22. Gilpin D, Coleman S, Hall S, Houston A, Karrasch J, Jones N. Injectable collagenase clostridium histolyticum: a new nonsurgical treatment for Dupuytren's disease. J Hand Surg Am. 2010;35(12):2027–38.
23. Nydick JA, Olliff BW, Garcia MJ, Hess AV, Stone JD. A comparison of percutaneous needle fasciotomy and collagenase injection for Dupuytren Disease. J Hand Surg Am. 2013;38(12):2377–80.
24. Chen NC, Shauver MJ, Chung KC. Cost-effectiveness of open partial fasciectomy, needle aponeurotomy and collagenase injection for Dupuytren Contracture. J Hand Surg. 2011;36A:1826–34.

25. McMillan C, Binhammer P. Steroid injection and needle aponeurotomy for Dupuytren contracture: a randomized, controlled study. J Hand Surg. 2012;37A:1307–12.
26. Hovius SE, Kan HJ, Smit X, Selles RW, Cardoso E, Khouri RK. Extensive percutaneous aponeurotomy and lipografting: a new treatment for Dupuytren disease. Plast Reconstr Surg. 2011;128:221–8.

Chapter 3
Ultrasound Assisted Needle Aponeurotomy in the Management of Dupuytren's Contracture

Vasileios I. Sakellariou and Marco Rizzo

Case Presentation

Herein, we present the case of a 75-years-old male—a retired sales engineer—with a 10-year history of progressive contracture of the ring finger of his dominant right hand. The chief complaint was a right ring finger contracture and diminished dexterity. The patient denied pain. However, he did have difficulty with activities such as putting on gloves and shaking hands, which worsened significantly over the last 2 years. He also complained of bilateral basal thumb pain and difficulty with grip related activities.

His medical history was positive for hypertension and ankle osteoarthritis. The surgical history included a laparoscopic cholecystectomy and an ankle arthrodesis. The patient received occasionally

V.I. Sakellariou, MD, MSc, PhD
Department of Orthopaedic Surgery, Attikon University Hospital,
1, Rimini Str, P.C. 124 62, Chaidari, Athens, Greece

M. Rizzo, MD (✉)
Department of Orthopedic Surgery, Division of Hand Surgery, Mayo Clinic,
200 First St. SW, Rochester, MN 55905, USA
e-mail: Rizzo.marco@mayo.edu

© Springer International Publishing Switzerland 2016   39
M. Rizzo (ed.), *Dupuytren's Contracture*,
DOI 10.1007/978-3-319-23841-8_3

nonsteroidal anti-inflammatory medication. The patient had a social history of occasional alcohol consumption. No known drug allergies were referred.

Diagnosis/Assessment

Physical exam revealed his grip strength to be 24 kg on the right, and 27 kg on the left side. Appositional pinch was 4.5 kg on the right, and 4 kg on the left hand; oppositional pinch was 5 kg on the right, and 4 kg on the left hand. Motion of his right hand at the ring finger was 63–100° at the metacarpophalangeal (MP) joint; proximal interphalangeal (PIP) hyperextended about 5°, and flexed to 115°. Distal interphalangeal (DIP) range of motion was 0–50°.

Wrist flexion was 60° and extension 70°, bilaterally. The patient had tenderness at the CMC joint bilaterally with a positive grind bilaterally. He had significant hyperextension of both MP joints. Palmar abduction of the thumb was 45° bilaterally and radial abduction was 30° bilaterally (Figs. 3.1 and 3.2).

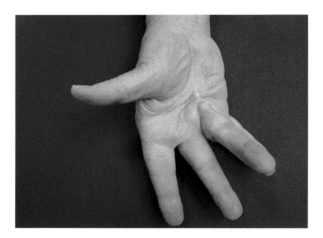

Fig. 3.1 Preoperative palmar view of the hand. Note the cord over the fourth MCP joint and the resulting contracture of the ring finger

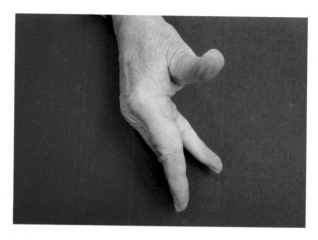

Fig. 3.2 Preoperative sagittal view of the hand showing the amount of the MCP extension deficit

Peripheral vascular examination showed an excellent cap refill. Neurologically, two-point discrimination using the Semmes-Weinstein monofilaments going from thumb to small finger was 6, 5, 5, 5, and 6 on the right, and 5, 5, 6, 6, and 6 on the left.

Radiographic evaluation revealed bilateral basal thumb arthritis and contracted ring finger, without obvious bony lesion in the fingers.

Management: Surgical Technique

Patient Information and Preoperative Evaluation

The patient was carefully evaluated before the procedure. Expectations were explained as possible improvement up to 90° of MCP and up to 50% improvement in PIP contracture [1]. After thorough clinical evaluation, the procedure was explained to the patient, including the importance of co-operation during surgical manipulations. The patient should be able to report paresthesias or numbness and avoid sudden movements. Potential complications (i.e., skin tear, nerve or tendon injury) and the significance to follow a postoperative care protocol were clearly explained and a written informed consent was received.

Procedure

The portals of fasciotomy were marked using a sterile marker pen (Fig. 3.3). Potential portals were considered areas where the skin is soft and the cord was a discrete linear structure that changed from soft to firm with joint extension. Firm nodules or deep impalpable cords were avoided because it is known that the associated risk for neurovascular damage is increased. Distance between portals was not closer than 5 mm. Portals were designed in line directly over the cord, and at its sides especially where its width exceeded 5 mm.

Ultrasound examination for preoperative mapping of spiral cords was performed prior to fasciotomy. The patient's hand was placed on the evaluation table palm up. Utilizing a Sonosite S-MSK series ultrasound machine in Doppler mode and 13–6 MHz hockey stick transducer, the arterial supply of the palm was evaluated and

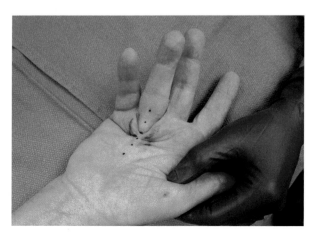

Fig. 3.3 Fasciotomy (needle stick sites) portals are planned and marked with a sterile marker pen

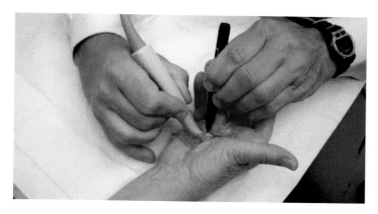

Fig. 3.4 The position of the superficial palmar arch is identified via Doppler and its position is recorded on the skin with an indelible skin marker

recorded. The position of the superficial palmar arch was identified via Doppler and its position was marked on the skin using an indelible skin marker (Fig. 3.4). The depth of the vascular supply was also noted. Via continued use of the Doppler, the common palmar digital arteries and proper palmar digital arteries were identified and superficially marked from the arch all the way to the PIP joint of the respective fingers (Figs. 3.5 and 3.6). Displacement of neurovascular structures associated with spiral cords were noted and marked.

Subsequently the palm and fingers were surgically prepped using chlorhexidine solution and drapped. Superficial pinpoint aliquots of 1 % lidocaine were intermittently injected over the pre-marked portals using a 30-gauge needle (Fig. 3.7). A fraction of one milliliter was utilized with each injection. The aim was to anesthetize the skin over the cord only and not the deeper digital nerves. Then a sterile short (0.75 in.) 19-gauge hollow needle was inserted perpendicular to the long axis of the cord fibers through anesthetic puncture sites. As one progresses into the finger a short (0.75 in.) 22 gauge needle was utilized. Using the digital nerve skin tracings as a guide, the needle was advanced to a depth of a few millimeters and carefully swept back and forth in a transverse orientation cutting the fibrotic bands (Fig. 3.8). The fascia was felt crisp or crunchy when being cut.

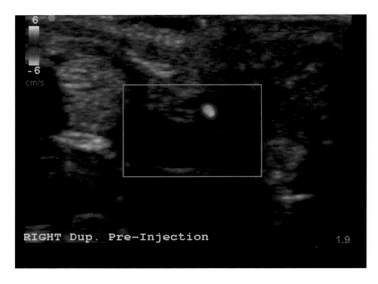

Fig. 3.5 Doppler image of digital artery with metacarpal on both sides

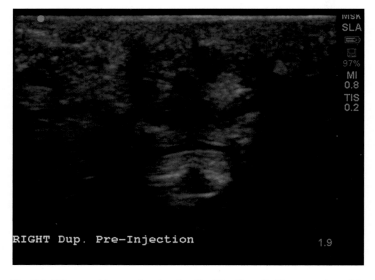

Fig. 3.6 Ultrasound image showing the identification of a Dupuytren's nodule

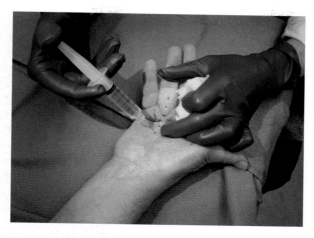

Fig. 3.7 Superficial pinpoint aliquots of 1 % lidocaine are intermittently injected over the pre-marked portals using a 30-gauge needle

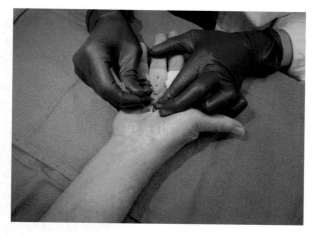

Fig. 3.8 Using the digital nerve skin tracings as a guide, the needle is advanced to a depth of a few millimeters and carefully swept back and forth in a transverse orientation cutting the fibrotic bands

Simultaneous passive cord tension was applied by holding the finger in extension during the procedure making the targeted cords more prominent and confirming contracture release. This process was repeated along the involved digit until optimal extension was attained. During the dissection of the fascial fibers flexor tendons were slack in order to reduce the risk of injury. Pressure on fingertips was avoided and the patient was reminded at that point to be calm trying to keep all fingers lax. The patient was queried routinely during the procedure to report "electrical-shock" sensations, which suggest that the needle was near or on a nerve. Fingertip sensitivity at both radial and ulnar sides of the digit was repeatedly checked through the procedure.

Tendon proximity was carefully and sequentially checked through the procedure. While the needle was inserted, the patient was asked to lightly flex and extend the PIP and DIP joints. Presence of needle motion demonstrated tendon penetration and was withdrawn. Bleeding at each needle site was controlled with pressure.

Releases were started at distal portals, progressing proximally. Passive stretching was done after each portal release as well as at the completion of all portals. During stretching patient's wrist was kept in flexion in order to prevent hyper-tensioning, which could eventually result in skin tear.

At the end of the procedure, portals and remaining nodules were injected with corticosteroids, and integrity of digital vessels was confirmed and documented with a final ultrasound scanning.

Post-procedure and Rehabilitation

Hemostasis was obtained with pressure. Small adhesive bandages (band-aids) were applied to the needle sites. Ice and elevation were recommended for the first 2 days while passive and active motions were allowed immediately (Figs. 3.9 and 3.10). Generally, the patient had no postoperative restrictions other than to avoid submerging his hands for 48 h.

The patient was instructed to use a daytime dynamic splint to help release residual contractures of the joints. It was recom-

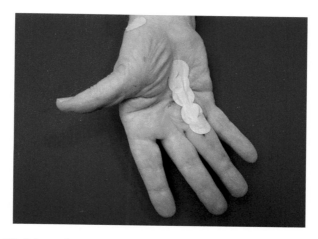

Fig. 3.9 Palmar view of the hand after the procedure. Note the correction of deformity and recovery of extension deficit of the ring finger

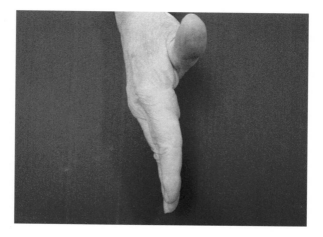

Fig. 3.10 Postoperative sagittal view of the hand showing all fingers in full extension

mended to utilize it for 30-min intervals three times per day (Fig. 3.11). A static extension (night) splints was also recommended and the patient was instructed to utilize it for 3 months postoperatively.

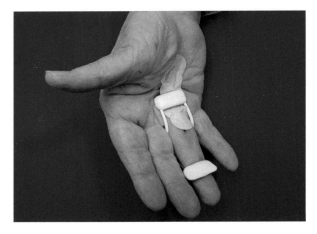

Fig. 3.11 A daytime dynamic splint is recommended to help release residual contractures of the joints

Potential Complications

Percutaneous needle fasciotomy is a safe minimally invasive procedure [2–4]. Recurrence of the disease is the most common complication after this procedure [5]. One should be aware that recurrence rate is higher compared to open procedures, and this is the reason that should be better limited to elderly, who want simple treatment without extensive wounds.

Damage to digital neurovascular structures is another potential complication [4, 5]. However, careful preoperative ultrasonographic mapping of the cords can diminish the possibilities of accidental lesions.

Skin tears and subsequent flexor tendon lesions are also possible [3, 4]. They usually occur in and adjacent to flexion creases at the PIP and the base of the finger. This is why skin creases should be better avoided during portal planning because of the proximity of the flexor sheath and the likelihood of skin tear. Once a tear develops, further attempts at passive extension are likely to propagate and thus are better avoided. Allowing a skin tear to first heal and then resuming NA is a reasonable course of action in these cases.

Literature Review

Dupuytren's contracture is a relatively common disorder that is characterized by a progressive fibrosis and thickening of the palmar fascia, and in long-standing or severe disease can result in shortening and thickening of the ligaments, as well as joint and skin contractures [6, 7]. Multiple etiologic factors can induce a pathognomonic fibroblastic proliferation and disorderly collagen deposition with fascial thickening and local formation of nodules and cords [6, 7].

Both conservative and surgical treatment modalities have been historically presented. Conservative measures include continuous slow skeletal traction, dimethyl sulfoxide, vitamin E, allopurinol, physical therapy, ultrasound therapy, glucocorticoid injections, interferon, and splinting, but are considered unsuccessful [8, 9]. Prophylactic external beam radiation therapy can prevent progression and provide symptomatic benefit in patients with mild to moderate flexion deformities [10]. Collagenase injection can be effective but limited to patients with less severe contractures (<50 % contracture) or early stages of the disease [11]. In addition, risks of allergic reaction, skin tearing, and immune response and tendon injury are associated with collagenase.

Surgical options include either fasciotomies (limited open or percutaneous), in which the cord is simply divided, or fasciectomies, in which the diseased fascia is excised [3, 6, 8, 12]. Selection of operative procedure is basically related to the severity of the disease and patient preference. Increasingly, patients express preference to avoid formal surgery for Dupuytren's. Tubiana grading system [13] encounters the amount of total passive extensive deficit (TPED) which is the sum of the passive extension deficits (PEDs) of the metacarpophalangeal (MCP), proximal interphalangeal (PIP), and distal interphalangeal (DIP) joints.

In general, percutaneous fasciotomies are best indicated for Tubiana grades I and II, but they are not as effective as limited open fasciotomies or fasciectomies for moderately severe forms of the disease (Tubiana stages III and IV). Treatment options include both surgical and conservative modalities.

Indications and Contraindications

It is generally agreed that percutaneous needle fasciotomy is best indicated for elderly patients with relatively mild contractures (Tubiana stages I and II) [4] especially with only a metacarpophalangeal deficit. Patients that need a stick or a palmar support to walk and those who have associated pathologies (arthrosis, short life expectancy) could benefit from this technique [4]. Relative indications could include patients willing to accept a higher risk of recurrence in the context of lower complication rates, faster recovery times, and minimal invasiveness [12]. Eaton presented four basic requirements for the procedure: (1) contracture due to a (2) palpable cord lying beneath (3) redundant skin in a (4) cooperative patient [1]. Other indications are more controversial; presence of algodystrophy, or patient who are very active and cannot take a sick leave are included in this group [2].

In contrary, percutaneous fasciotomies should not be attempted in the absence of a palpable cord and they should not be expected to correct longitudinally inadequate skin or scars [4]. While debatable, infiltrating disease, inaccessible multiple cords, postsurgical digital recurrences in young adults, and severe and long present digital disease causing the stiffness of the PIP joint are reported as clear contraindications by Foucher et al. [2]. This technique is also less effective for contractures not resulting from Dupuytren's disease or for patients with constitutionally treatment resistant disease. Rijssen et al. showed that percutaneous needle fasciotomy is not effective as limited open fasciotomy for Tubiana stages III and IV and thus these cases should be considered as relative contraindications [4]. It is debatable if use of anticoagulant drugs is a contraindication [14] or actually a relative indication of the procedure compared to limited open fasciotomy or fasciectomy [1, 2].

The main advantages of fasciotomies are lower incidence of nerve injury, flare reaction, and reflex sympathetic dystrophy as well as decreased time needed for recovery [3, 4]. Needle percutaneous fasciotomies can be performed in the office setting, usually permit return to normal manual activities within a week after the procedure. They are gaining popularity due to the growing demand for fast recovery, low complication rate, and minimal invasiveness, which allows both hands to be treated on consecutive days when needed. Chen et al. also showed that this is a cost-effective procedure over open procedures [15].

The main disadvantage is a higher recurrence rate compared to limited open fasciotomies and fasciectomies that occur more rapidly [4]. Moreover, the procedure may be limited only for contractures that they do not include severe skin shortage or capsular shrinkage of the proximal interphalangeal (PIP) joint [1].

Clinical Pearls/Pitfalls

- It is a straightforward procedure.
- Combines the advantages of a minimally invasive procedure with the increased safety of the ultrasonographic mapping of the digital neurovascular bundles.
- Lowering the small, but significant, risk of postoperative finger numbness with preoperative ultrasound mapping is reasonable in our view.
- Ultrasound mapping does increase procedure cost but is favorably received by patients, as it likely reduces their surgical risk without adding discomfort.

References

1. Eaton C. Percutaneous fasciotomy for Dupuytren's contracture. J Hand Surg. 2011;36(5):910.
2. Foucher G, Medina J, Navarro R. Percutaneous needle aponeurotomy. Complications and results. Chirurgie de la main. 2001;20(3):206.
3. Rahr L, Sondergaard P, Bisgaard T, Baad-Hansen T. Percutaneous needle fasciotomy for primary Dupuytren's contracture. J Hand Surg Eur Vol. 2011;36(7):548.
4. van Rijssen AL, ter Linden H, Werker PM. Five-year results of a randomized clinical trial on treatment in Dupuytren's disease: percutaneous needle fasciotomy versus limited fasciectomy. Plast Reconstr Surg. 2012; 129(2):469.
5. Rayan GM. Dupuytren's disease: anatomy, pathology, presentation, and treatment. Instr Course Lect. 2007;56:101.

6. Trojian TH, Chu SM. Dupuytren's disease: diagnosis and treatment. Am Fam Physician. 2007;76(1):86.

7. Townley WA, Baker R, Sheppard N, Grobbelaar AO. Dupuytren's contracture unfolded. BMJ. 2006;332(7538):397.

8. Rayan GM. Dupuytren disease: anatomy, pathology, presentation, and treatment. J Bone Joint Surg Am. 2007;89(1):189.

9. Hurst LC, Badalamente MA. Nonoperative treatment of Dupuytren's disease. Hand Clin. 1999;15(1):97.

10. Seegenschmiedt MH, Olschewski T, Guntrum F. Radiotherapy optimization in early-stage Dupuytren's contracture: first results of a randomized clinical study. Int J Radiat Oncol Biol Phys. 2001;49(3):785.

11. Hurst LC, Badalamente MA, Hentz VR, Hotchkiss RN, Kaplan FT, Meals RA, Smith TM, Rodzvilla J. Injectable collagenase clostridium histolyticum for Dupuytren's contracture. N Engl J Med. 2009;361(10):968.

12. van Rijssen AL, Gerbrandy FS, Ter Linden H, Klip H, Werker PM. A comparison of the direct outcomes of percutaneous needle fasciotomy and limited fasciectomy for Dupuytren's disease: a 6-week follow-up study. J Hand Surg. 2006;31(5):717.

13. Tubiana R. The cutaneous stage in the surgical treatment of Dupuytren's disease. Ann Chir Plast. 1963;8:157.

14. Symes T, Stothard J. Two significant complications following percutaneous needle fasciotomy in a patient on anticoagulants. J Hand Surg. 2006;31(6):606.

15. Chen NC, Shauver MJ, Chung KC. Cost-effectiveness of open partial fasciectomy, needle aponeurotomy, and collagenase injection for dupuytren contracture. J Hand Surg. 1826;36(11):2011.

Chapter 4
Corticosteroid Injections and Needle Aponeurotomy in the Management of Dupuytren's Contracture

Paul Binhammer

Case Presentation

A 59-year-old right hand dominant female bookkeeper presented with concerns about Dupuytren's disease of her right small finger. She had noticed this for 3–4 years. She had a family history of Dupuytren's disease. She was otherwise well. She was on no medications. Clinical examination revealed a right small finger PIP flexion deformity of 57°. She had an ulnar-sided cord. The patient was informed of the underlying pathophysiology and the variable progression of Dupuytren's disease. She was informed of her options for management including surgical excision and percutaneous release. She was informed of average success and failure rates and warned of the risk of infection and numbness. The requirement for splinting and therapy was explained. She decided to proceed with percutaneous release.

P. Binhammer, MD, FRCS(C) (✉)
Hand Wrist and Microvascular Surgery, Sunnybrook Health Sciences Centre, 2075 Bayview Ave, Toronto, ON, Canada, M4N 3M5
e-mail: p.binhammer@utoronto.ca

© Springer International Publishing Switzerland 2016

M. Rizzo (ed.), *Dupuytren's Contracture*,
DOI 10.1007/978-3-319-23841-8_4

Management

Under alcohol prep using 1 % lidocaine and 0.5 % bupivacaine with epinephrine, for local infiltration, she underwent routine release of her right small finger to complete release using the technique described below. The release was performed at multiple levels. She had steroid injection of 0.5 cc of triamcinolone 40. She was referred to the therapist for a splint to maintain the digit in extension. The splint was to be worn at night. There was no therapy program.

Six weeks following the procedure she returned to have 0.4 cc of triamcinolone 40 injected along the length of the prior cord. The patient was advised to continue splinting for another 6 weeks at night.

At 3 and 6 months post-procedure the patient was measured to have a straight digit.

Outcome

The patient returned 5 years later with recurrent contracture of the right small finger. She had a precentral cord with an MP contracture of 50° and PIP of 78°. After reviewing the available options including surgery, needle aponeurotomy and collagenase and their advantages, disadvantages, risks and benefits, she elected to undergo needle aponeurotomy. She underwent repeat needle aponeurotomy with steroid injection to achieve a straight digit (Figs. 4.1, 4.2, and 4.3). She was referred for splinting.

Literature Review

Needle aponeurotomy (NA) has the benefits when treating Dupuytren's disease of a rapid recovery and low risk of complications, which include tendon rupture and/or laceration, nerve injury, and infection [1, 2]. Reported recurrence rates range from 33 to 100 % [3, 4].

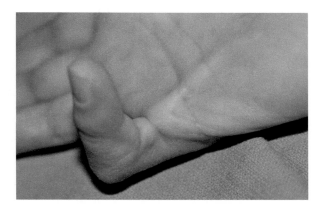

Fig. 4.1 Patient with right hand small finger Dupuytren's cord with significant contracture

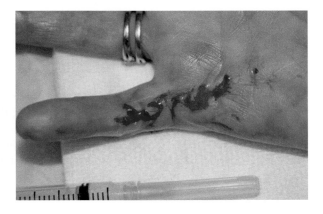

Fig. 4.2 Photo of finger following needle aponeurotomy

Triamcinolone acetonide injections have been used to treat keloids and hypertrophic scars with success [5]. Triamcinolone has also been used to alter disease progression of Dupuytren's nodules [6].

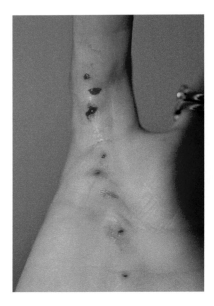

Fig. 4.3 Photo following injection of triamcinolone

Technique

The combination of NA and triamcinolone can be used together in the treatment of Dupuytren's disease [7]. Under local anaesthesia using 1 % lidocaine and alcohol skin preparation, the cord is percutaneously divided using the bevel of a 16-gauge injection needle. Local anaesthesia is restricted to the skin and a digital nerve block is avoided so that any contact between the releasing needle and the neurovascular bundle can be identified. Multiple points of division are performed along the length of the cord. The procedure is terminated when the finger can be passively straightened to an extended posture, to a total extension deficit of 0. If the digit can not be straightened, further points of release are performed until the digit can be straightened or it is felt there are no more points that can be released. Supplemental digital block is performed at this point using a long-acting local anaesthetic to provide the patient with post-operative anaesthesia. Closed manipulation can be performed at this point. A 25-gauge needle is used to administer injections of triamcinolone directly into the cords causing contracture immediately following PNA. The point of injections is between the points of release. The preparation used is Triamcinolone Acetonide Injectable Suspension USP (40 mg/ml). The amount injected is approximately 1 cc per digit divided between the release points. The triamcinolone suspension leaks out through the holes of the NA. A bandage or small dressing is applied and usually discontinued within 48 h. No medications are prescribed. Patients are fitted with a custom thermoplastic orthosis and are directed to wear it at night for 3 months to maintain digital extension. A daily stretching program is advised for the first 6 weeks in order to maintain range of motion. Patients are not followed by a therapist.

Follow-up injections of triamcinolone are given at 6 weeks and 3 months to areas of palpable thickness along previously released cords. If no area of palpable thickness is present, no injection is administered. Injections are not administered to newly developed cords. The triamcinolone dose is split between injection sites. The amount injected at 6 weeks is less than 1 cc per digit and at 3 months this is approximately 0.5 cc.

Results

A randomized trial was performed following NA-treated patients with or without a series of triamcinolone injections and compared total active extension deficit (TAED) [7]. The study involved 47 patients. Correction at 6 months was 87 % of pre-operative TAED for the TA group versus 64 % for the control group. This difference was statistically significant. The amount of triamcinolone administered did not correlate with TAED improvement. PIP joint correction was statistically better for the triamcinolone group at all time points measured, 6 weeks, 3 months and 6 months. There were no adverse outcomes associated with the administration of triamcinolone.

A follow-up study looking at the same group of patients found that mean TAED was significantly less in the triamcinolone group between 13 and 24 months but not at 36 months [8]. Kaplan-Meier survival estimates demonstrated a significantly higher percentage of NA without triamcinolone patients expected to return for retreatment by 24 but not by 36 months. Younger age, more than one joint treated at the initial NA, and TAED severity throughout the follow-up period were associated with earlier retreatment.

References

1. Eaton C. Percutaneous fasciotomy for Dupuytren's contracture. J Hand Surg Am. 2011;36(5):910–5.
2. Foucher G, Medina J, Navarro R. Percutaneous needle aponeurotomy: complications and results. J Hand Surg Br. 2003;28(5):427–31.
3. van Rijssen AL, ter Linden H, Werker PMN. Five-year results of a randomized clinical trial on treatment in Dupuytren's disease: percutaneous needle fasciotomy versus limited fasciectomy. Plast Reconstr Surg. 2012; 129(2):469–77.
4. Werker PMN, Pess GM, van Rijssen AL, Denkler K. Correction of contracture and recurrence rates of Dupuytren contracture following invasive treatment: the importance of clear definitions. J Hand Surg Am. 2012;37(10): 2095–105.
5. Ketchum LD, Robinson DW, Masters FW. Follow-up on treatment of hypertrophic scars and keloids with triamcinolone. Plast Reconstr Surg. 1971;48(3):256–9.
6. Ketchum LD, Donahue TK. The injection of nodules of Dupuytren's disease with triamcinolone acetonide. J Hand Surg Am. 2000;25(6):1157–62.
7. McMillan C, Binhammer P. Steroid injection and needle aponeurotomy for Dupuytren contracture: a randomized, controlled study. J Hand Surg Am. 2012;37(7):1307–12.
8. McMillan C, Binhammer P. Steroid injection and needle aponeurotomy for Dupuytren contracture: long term follow-up of a randomized, controlled study. J Hand Surg Am. 2014;39(10):1942–7.

Chapter 5

Clostridial Collagenase Injections in the Treatment of Dupuytren's Contracture

Jan-Ragnar Haugstvedt

Case Presentation

An 84-year-old right-hand dominant man, previously engineer, showed up in the clinic and asked for advice for treatment of his flexed fingers. He was being treated for hypertension, was on salicylic acid, and had twice been in surgery due to a colon cancer. Following the last surgery 4 years ago, the follow-ups had shown no signs of recurrence of his cancer. His current problem was his right hand. He was no longer able to shake hands with people, he had problems grasping an object, and the fingers "were in the way." The flexed position of his fingers had gradually progressed during the last 2 years. He was familiar with the condition as he had seen several other family members with a somewhat similar appearance of their hands, and he had been surfing the Internet looking for different possibilities for treatment.

J.-R. Haugstvedt, MD, PhD (✉)
Department of Orthopedics, Østfold Hospital Trust,
Peer Gynts vei 78, 1575 Moss, Norway
e-mail: jrhaugstvedt@gmail.com

© Springer International Publishing Switzerland 2016
M. Rizzo (ed.), *Dupuytren's Contracture*,
DOI 10.1007/978-3-319-23841-8_5

59

Diagnosis/Assessment

The patient was found to have the following changes in his right
hand: In his ring finger he had a 70° contracture over his metacarpophalangeal (MCP) joint while his proximal interphalangeal
(PIP) joint was in an 80° flexed position (Figs. 5.1 and 5.2). He
demonstrated a cord running from the proximal part of the palm of
the hand to the middle phalanx of his ring finger. There was an
involvement of the little finger as this finger was somewhat
adducted and flexed; however no separate palpable cord was running from the palm of the hand to this finger.

The changes found in his hand were found to be "classical" for
the changes seen in a patient with a Dupuytren's contracture, and
as already mentioned he was well aware of the diagnosis before his
visit. He was informed about the disease, the different changes that
could be found in the different fascias in different parts of the body,
and he was informed about different forms of treatment. With the
changes described, there was a clear indication for treatment. The
patient being in the mid-80s, and already having had some major

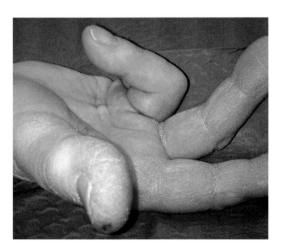

Fig. 5.1 The right hand before collagenase injection showing the flexed fourth
finger with the cord running from the palm of the hand towards the finger itself

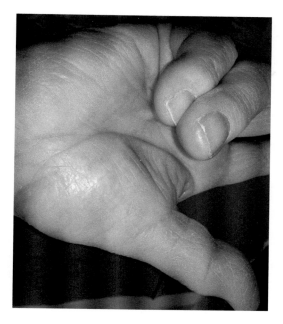

Fig. 5.2 A view from the volar side of the hand showing that the fifth finger also has a flexed position before treatment

surgery for other conditions, was not interested in any kind of surgery. He felt he would have a better quality of life if he only would be able to straighten his fingers a little more and he asked for injection treatment.

Management

The patient, who was not allergic to any specific drugs and had not received any Tetracycline antibiotics the last 14 days prior to treatment, had an injection of collagenase (Xiapex®) in his hand. The localization of the injection in the cord was between the distal crease of the palm of the hand and the proximal phalanx. The patient did not experience any pain, waited at the office for half an hour (for a potential allergic reaction), and went home.

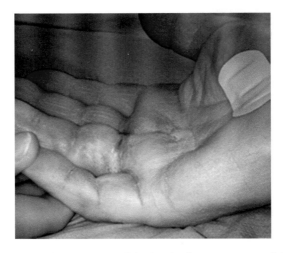

Fig. 5.3 The day after collagenase injection the fingers were extended. Notice the superficial rupture of the skin at the base of the fourth finger as well as the edema and the bleeding in the soft tissue

The patient returned the next day and reported no pain or discomfort, although some edema of his hand was noted. After local anesthesia had been given, the fingers were extended. A clear sound was heard when the cord ruptured. The fingers were passively extended; however it was neither possible to have full extension in either of the affected fingers nor in the different joints of the fourth finger. There was a rupture of the superficial layer of the skin; however there was no deep wound that required any specific form of treatment (Fig. 5.3). A splint was adapted and the patient was asked to use this as a night splint for the following 3 months (Fig. 5.4).

Outcome

Ten weeks after treatment the patient reported on a good result (Figs. 5.5 and 5.6). Even though he was not able to fully extend his finger, his quality of life had improved; he was able to shake hands

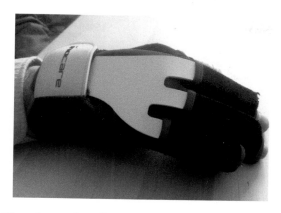

Fig. 5.4 The patient used a splint during nighttime for 3 months following the injection treatment

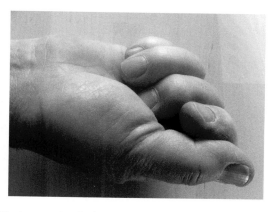

Fig. 5.5 Maximum active flexion 10 weeks after treatment with collagenase

with people, to grasp an object, and to wash his face using his hands. Two years after treatment he was still happy with the result. Using a Visual Analog Scale he reported 8 (0 being "worst" outcome, while 10 was "perfect"). The reason why he was not totally satisfied was due to the little finger, which, previously was without any cord and had not been treated, had started to flex. The situation,

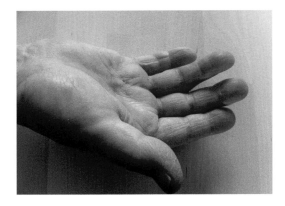

Fig. 5.6 Maximum active extension 10 weeks after treatment with collagenase

though, was not so bad that he considered another treatment; however he stated that he would have done the same procedure over again and would ask for another injection if the situation evolved and he would need treatment.

Literature Review

In one epidemiologic study from Iceland [1] 19.2% of men and 4.4% of women showed signs of Dupuytren's contracture, the prevalence increasing with age, the highest value found in men between 70 and 74 years old. Thus for surgeons working in Scandinavia treatment of the so-called Viking disease is common. I have performed needle aponeurotomy, open fasciectomy with or without excision of overlying skin (with skin transplant if necessary), I have performed microvascular free tissue transfer to cover the defect after resection of the changes, and I've done arthrodesis of a joint, or partial or ray amputation of an affected finger. Thus I had a variety of appliances in my toolbox, and however still could need yet another one for selected cases.

I heard about collagenase in the late 1990s [2]; however it took some years before papers describing the effect of the treatment were published [3, 4]. In the first papers it was reported that contractures of the finger joints were corrected after collagenase injections while patients treated with placebo did not achieve the same corrections and did not have the same improvements in range of motion.

In a study based on 11 clinical trials ($n = 1082$), the investigators found the incidence of adverse events (nerve injury, neurapraxia, CRPS, and arterial injury) was lower with collagenase injection compared with complications from fasciectomy [5]. Tendon injury, skin injury, and hematoma occurred more often with collagenase. Other side effects experienced with collagenase included pain at the injection site, edema, some pain in the extremity, and lymphadenopathy. These changes were all transient.

Even though fasciectomy may still be considered the gold standard for treatment of Dupuytren's disease, needle aponeurotomy or collagenase injections are widely used. The patients seeking for advice and help are today better educated than years ago and have very often been searching the Internet for the kind of treatment they want [6]. They ask for a specific treatment, and we, as doctors, have to decide the proper, or best treatment for the patient; however there should be the same indication for treatment whatever treatment method is being used.

Patients have often specific problems that lead them to the doctor asking for treatment, the most common problems being "difficulty washing self," "difficulty picking things up," and "finger hooking on things" [7]. The authors state that the long-term outcome of treatment may be more important than quick recovery to patients.

For the first patients treated with collagenase injections, it was advocated to treat one cord affecting one joint at a time. In the last years, however, there have been trials on injections into cords affecting two joints at the same time. The results of one multicenter study showed effective treatment with 76% clinical success for treatment of MCP joints and 33% for PIP joints. 60% of the patients in this multicenter study were very satisfied with treatment, although the patients experienced more pain in the extremity and local edema, all of the symptoms being transient [8]. Treatment of more than one joint or two cords at the same time is gaining popularity.

For a long time Food and Drug Association approved maximum injections of 0.58 mg of the enzyme into one cord at a time. However later studies have been performed using 0.78 mg of the enzyme at one time, "the entire bottle," allowing the doctor to give multiple injections into several cords using the so-called slow intracord multi-cord (SIMple) technique [9]. The results reported in this one study were comparable with previously published studies using a lower dose. The author suggests that using this method there could be healthcare savings compared with other type of treatments as the patient would not have to return for another later injection or surgery.

While considering using collagenase injections, one may wonder if it's possible to use this technique in patients that had previous surgery for Dupuytren's disease. In one paper, data from 12 clinical trials where collagenase had been used were pooled and evaluated [10]. Some of the patients included in the study had injection of collagenase in a previously nonoperated hand, while other patients had previous surgery in the hand where they now had injections. The authors did neither find any differences in reduction of the flexion contractures of the finger joints, nor in the improvements of the range of motion between the two groups, and both groups of patients were equally satisfied with the treatment. The adverse events (injection site hemorrhage, blood blister, axillary peripheral edema, contusion, pain in the extremity, tenderness, ecchymosis, and lymphadenopathy) varied between the groups; however none were clinically relevant. The authors conclude that injection treatment with collagenase is also well tolerated in patients previously surgically treated for Dupuytren's disease in the same finger.

If the treatment with collagenase is not successful, there might be a demand for later surgery. In one study [11], the authors report on the surgical findings after initial treatment with collagenase. Nine surgeons reported on a total of 15 patients with surgical treatment following previous collagenase injections. In 9 out of 15 cases the surgery was considered as easier or equivalent to a primary operation, 2 as equivalent to and 4 as harder than a revision operation. The problems faced were abnormal thickening and adherence of the cord with changes of the anatomy and troublesome dissection. I have performed surgery in one case myself without having any problems with the dissection of the anatomical structures.

It is difficult to have one good outcome measure to evaluate the results after treatment for Dupuytren's disease. There should probably be a set of validated outcome measures to monitor the natural history of the disease as well as compare between treatment modalities [12]. Patient Related Outcome Measure (PROM) has been used; however the question is if this correlates with the patient's quality of life (QoL) [13]. Tests that have been used include Disability of Arm, Shoulder and Hand (DASH), the URAM scale (Unité Rhumatologique des Affections de la Main), Southampton Dupuytren's Scoring Scheme (SDSS) as well as the Michigan Hand Questionnaire (MHQ); however even if at least some of the tests are meant specifically for Dupuytren's disease, none seem to be working very well. VAS could be used to reflect change in the symptom of pain over time in an individual; it has good intra-rater reliability and can be used to distinguish between any specific treatment satisfaction being used and the treatment outcome [14].

Clinical Pearls and Pitfalls

- The same indications should be used for treatment of Dupuytren's disease regardless of what treatment modality is being used.
- Clostridial Collagenase injections could be used for one cord in one finger affecting one joint, however have also been shown to be effective if using multiple injections affecting several cords/joints.
- When injecting the collagenase, the needle should be directed away from the flexor tendon in order to avoid the risk of flexor tendon rupture; the needle should come from dorsal to volar or pass through the skin in an oblique manner with the needle pointing beside the tendon.

- Edema and bleeding are often seen after treatment with collagenase; thus caution is necessary when the patient is taking any anticoagulants.
- Collagenase can be used for recurrences of Dupuytren's disease; however it is not indicated for treatment of scar tissue.

References

1. Gudmundsson KG. Epidemiology of Dupuytren's disease: clinical, serological, and social assessment The Reykjavik Study. J Clin Epidemiol. 2000;53(3):291–6.
2. Starkweather KD, Lattuga S, Hurst LC, Badalamente MA, Guilak F, Sampson SP, Dowd A, Wisch D. Collagenase in the treatment of Dupuytren's disease: an in vitro study. J Hand Surg Am. 1996;21(3): 490–5.
3. Badalamente MA, Hurst LC. Efficacy and safety of injectable mixed collagenase subtypes in the treatment of Dupuytren's contracture. J Hand Surg Am. 2007;32(6):767–74.
4. Hurst LC, Badalamente MA, Hentz VR, Hotchkiss RN, Kaplan FT, Meals RA, Smith TM, Rodzvilla J, CORD I Study Group. Injectable collagenase clostridium histolyticum for Dupuytren's contracture. N Engl J Med. 2009;361(10):968–79.
5. Peimer CA, Wilbrand S, Gerber RA, Chapman D, Szczypa PP. Safety and tolerability of collagenase Clostridium histolyticum and fasciectomy for Dupuytren's contracture. J Hand Surg. 2015;40(2):141–9.
6. Hentz VR. Collagenase injections for treatment of Dupuytren disease. Hand Clin. 2014;30(1):25–32.
7. Rodrigues JN, Zhang W, Scammell BD, Davis TR. What patients want from the treatment of Dupuytren's disease-is the Unité Rhumatologique de Affections de la Main (URAM) scale relevant? J Hand Surg Eur. 2015;40(2):150–4.
8. Coleman S, Gilpin D, Kaplan FT, Houston A, Kaufman GJ, Cohen BM, Jones N, Tursi JP. Efficacy and safety of concurrent collagenase clostridium histolyticum injections for multiple Dupuytren contractures. J Hand Surgery Am. 2014;39(1):57–64.
9. Verheyden JR. Early outcomes of a sequential series of 144 patients with Dupuytren's contracture treated by collagenase injection using an increased dose, multi-cord technique. J Hand Surg Eur. 2015;40(2):133–40.
10. Bainbridge C, Gerber RA, Szczypa PP, Smith T, Kushner H, Cohen B, Hellio Le Graverand-Gastineau MP. Efficacy of collagenase in patients who did and did not have previous hand surgery for Dupuytren's contracture. J Plast Surg Hand Surg. 2012;46(3–4):177–83.

11. Hay DC, Louie DL, Earp BE, Kaplan FT, Akelman E, Blazar PE. Surgical findings in the treatment of Dupuytren's disease after initial treatment with clostridial collagenase. J Hand Surg Eur. 2014;39(5):463–5.
12. Ball C, Pratt AL, Nanchahal J. Optimal functional outcome measures for assessing treatment for Dupuytren's disease: a systematic review and recommendations for future practice. BMC Musculoskelet Disord. 2013;14:131.
13. Wilburn J, McKenna SP, Perry-Hinsley D, Bayat A. The Impact of Dupuytren disease on patient activity and quality of life. J Hand Surg. 2013;38(6):1209–14.
14. Badalamente M, Coffelt L, Elfar J, Gaston G, Hammert W, Huang J, Lattanza L, Macdermid J, Merrell G, Netscher D, Panthaki Z, Rafijah G, Trczinski D, Graham B. American Society for Surgery of the Hand Clinical Trials and Outcomes Committee. Measurement scales in clinical research of the upper extremity, part 2: outcome measures in studies of the hand/wrist and shoulder/elbow. J Hand Surg Am. 2013;38(2):407–12.

Suggested Readings

Atroshi I, Strandberg E, Lauritzson A, Ahlgren E, Waldén M. Costs for collagenase injections compared with fasciectomy in the treatment of Dupuytren's contracture: a retrospective cohort study. BMJ Open. 2014;15(4):e004166. doi:10.1136/bmjopen-2013-004166.
McGrouther DA, Jenkins A, Brown S, Gerber RA, Szczypa P, Cohen B. The efficacy and safety of collagenase clostridium histolyticum in the treatment of patients with moderate Dupuytren's contracture. Curr Med Res Opin. 2014;30(4):733–9.
Mickelson DT, Noland SS, Watt AJ, Kollitz KM, Vedder NB, Huang JI. Prospective randomized controlled trial comparing 1. versus 7-day manipulation following collagenase injection for dupuytren contracture. J Hand Surgery Am. 2014;39(10):1933–41.
Peimer CA, Blazar P, Coleman S, Kaplan FT, Smith T, Tursi JP, Cohen B, Kaurman GJ, Lindau T. Dupuytren contracture recurrence following treatment with collagenase clostridium histolyticum (CORDLESS study): 3-year data. J Hand Surg Am. 2013;38(1):12–22.

Chapter 6
Minimally Invasive Partial Fasciectomy

Sidney M. Jacoby and Justin D. Stull

Case Presentation

A 76-year-old man presented to our clinic with complaints of decreased right hand function resulting from a flexion deformity to his right fourth digit, with increasing severity over the past several years. His past medical history was significant for medically controlled hypertension, controlled type II diabetes mellitus, and benign prostatic hypertrophy. His past surgical history was unremarkable and limited to cataract removal. His review of systems was noncontributory. The patient was of Irish decent. He reported one sibling, a brother who died at 67, whose hand also

S.M. Jacoby, MD
Department of Orthopaedic Surgery, Thomas Jefferson University Hospital,
The Philadelphia Hand Center, PC, The Franklin, 834 Chestnut Street,
Suite G114, Philadelphia, PA 19107, USA
e-mail: smjacoby@handcenters.com

J.D. Stull, BA (✉)
Sidney Kimmel Medical College at Thomas Jefferson University,
Thomas Jefferson University Hospital, 1015 Walnut Street,
Philadelphia, PA 19107, USA
e-mail: Justin.stull@gmail.com

© Springer International Publishing Switzerland 2016
M. Rizzo (ed.), *Dupuytren's Contracture*,
DOI 10.1007/978-3-319-23841-8_6

"clawed up" as he aged. The patient was a retired construction worker, married, without children. He was a non-smoker, non-drug user, but enjoyed a drink with dinner. He reported no known food or drug allergies.

Physical Assessment and Diagnosis

Visual inspection of the patient's affected hand revealed obvious contractures of the right fourth finger at both the MCP and PIP joints. A stout, pretendinous cord along the ray of the ring finger with adjacent pitting at the distal palmar crease was observed. On palpation, the stout cord was easily appreciated from the medial aspect of the thenar crease to the base of the fourth MCP joint. There were no palpable nodules. No pain or tenderness was noted on deep palpation of the cords. Using a handheld goniometer, the measured MCP joint contracture was 40°. Holding the MCP joint in neutral, the contracture of the PIP joint was measured to be 80°.

Dupuytren's disease most commonly involves the fourth digit, and the MCP is the most often involved joint [1]. The highest prevalence of Dupuytren's disease is among 50–70-year-old males of North European decent, including those of Irish heritage, such as the patient in this vignette [1, 2]. Autosomal dominant genetic inheritance has been reported as a major risk factor for increased predisposition to the disease. Further, it is thought that microvascular disease and myofibroblast proliferation play an important role in disease presentation and progression; smoking, diabetes, repetitive trauma, advanced age, male sex, and alcohol consumption have all been linked as contributors to this pathogenesis [1, 3–6].

Histology can be useful to gauge the severity of the disease; however Dupuytren's contracture remains a clinical diagnosis; therefore, imaging and biopsies are not routinely conducted to confirm diagnosis.

Management Options

In patients with MCP joint contracture >30°, PIP joint contracture >30°, or any patient who presents with functional disability, surgical management is appropriate. Patients without advanced disease and those patients who demonstrate a normal "table–top test" can be treated with expectant observation.

Nonsurgical options, including percutaneous needle aponeurectomy (PNA), have reported early results comparable to some standard fasciectomy techniques. Lower rates of long-term success and diminished visualization of critical structures during the procedure are two potential drawbacks to PNA, which is usually reserved for those with total contractures of <90° [1, 7–10]. Another nonsurgical option, collagenase injection, has yielded good preliminary outcomes, especially in patients with less severe contractures, but sufficient long-term analysis is pending. One potential drawback to collagenase is its cost, and in certain circumstances difficulty in obtaining expedient insurance clearance [11–14].

Primary surgical options vary by the invasiveness, and the extent of excised tissue, which commonly revolves around the pattern of palmar fascia involvement. At one end of the spectrum exists the minimally invasive partial fasciectomy, which utilizes multiple small transverse incisions to remove diseased fascial cords [10, 15, 16], and at the other end is the open radical fasciectomy, which has generally fallen out of favor due to its increased morbidity and lengthy recovery time [1, 17, 18]. Between the two ends of the surgical spectrum exists options that differ in the degree of tissue excision and the pattern of exposure. For primary surgical procedures in the absence of diathesis, preference for minimally invasive surgical management allows for a quick return to activity, less morbidity than more extensive techniques, and preservation of facial planes that still allows for future revision procedures if necessary.

Management Chosen

Minimally invasive partial fasciectomy with multiple transverse incisions was performed.

Clinical Course and Outcome

With the patient under general anesthesia, a pneumatic tourniquet was applied, prior to skin incision. One-centimeter transverse incisions were made along the length of the pretendinous cord beginning at the proximal palmar crease, extending to the PIP joint (Fig. 6.1). Hemostasis was achieved through the use of bipolar electrocautery, and special attention was given to identifying and isolating neurovascular bundles with reverse Hohmann retractors. With this approach 1–2 cm longitudinal cord segments were excised through each transverse incision in a proximal to distal manner (Fig. 6.2). Even with isolation of the neurovascular bundles, resection of retrovascular cords must be done with great caution as digital neurovascular bundles may be displaced central, proximal, or superficial, particularly at the level of palmar-digital crease. If visualization is not possible, the cord release must be forgone to judicially protect the neurovasculature. One benefit of this technique is that it allows for extension of the incisions and conversion to open fasciectomy if necessary. Once cord release is complete, and the affected digit was able to achieve maximum extension on passive manipulation, closure was completed with 4-0 nylon sutures, and a soft dressing applied (Fig. 6.3).

At 1-week follow-up our patient had his surgical dressings removed, with evidence of excellent early healing. He was maintained in an extension splint and instructed to begin active range of motion exercises for the wrist and digits. Sutures were removed at the 10-day postoperative marker, with continuation of splinting, range of motion exercise, and instruction for scar massage. Strengthening began at postoperative week 4 with return to daily activity at week 6.

Review of Literature and Discussion

Widely accepted guidelines for treatment of Dupuytren's disease stipulate that surgical management should be sought for individuals with >30° flexion contracture of the MCP and >10–15° flexion

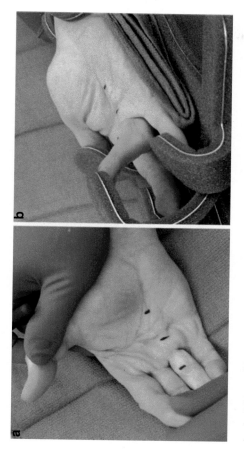

Fig. 6.1 Preoperative incision markings. (**a**) *Frontal plane*: 1 cm transverse incision markings are made 2–3 cm apart moving distally from the proximal palmar crease, approaching the PIP joint. (**b**) *Oblique plane*: Surgical positions demonstrate disease of the MCP joint and PIP joint of 40° and 80° respectively

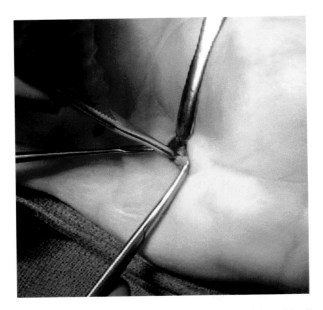

Fig. 6.2 Intraoperative photograph. Image illustrates the excision of the diseased Dupuytren's cord from a segment distal to the transverse incision

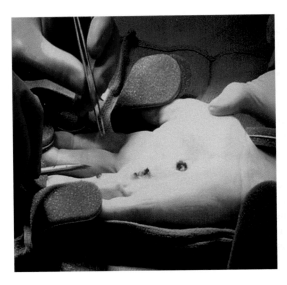

Fig. 6.3 Intraoperative photograph. Following excision of all diseased Dupuytren's cord through multiple transverse incisions, complete extension is achieved at both the MCP and PIP joints

contracture of the PIP [1, 8]. The literature, however, is inconclusive with regard to which technique is the preferred primary treatment option [19]. Most commonly, the extent of disease and likelihood for recurrence drives decision making. The patient in this case is clearly a surgical candidate (MCP flexion of 40° with PIP involvement) with many risk factors for recurrence and mild to moderate disease, but also presents at a late age without disease diathesis, therefore allowing for consideration of a wide range of treatment intervention options.

A variety of dermal incision patterns have been described with varying degrees of fasciectomies. Transverse incisions have been proposed to limit tissue disruption through maximally preserved blood supply, and minimal tension exertion on the dermis as compared to longitudinal incisions [20–22]. As a result, transverse incisions have been incorporated into a number of fasciectomy techniques to reduce the likelihood of recurrent disease. Minimally invasive partial fasciectomy utilizes multiple small transverse incisions, sequentially spaced along pathologic cords, through which the fasciectomy is subcutaneously performed proximally and distally to remove the diseased tissue without substantial incision [10]. By avoiding a large incision and associated traumatic inflammatory response running in parallel with the diseased fascia, minimally invasive partial fasciectomy offers a less invasive procedure with quick return to activity and good outcomes with appropriate patient selection [10, 15, 16]. To a great extent, this procedure also maintains fascial planes, which is of great importance should revision procedures become necessary in the future. With 2-year follow-up, several studies have reported outcomes on par with other minimally invasive techniques including sustained MCP flexion correction at final data collection [10, 16]. One 2-year follow-up reported no recurrences [16], and a second study with average follow-up of 15 months reported complete resolution of PIP joint contracture in a small cohort. [15] Another study, with a starting $n = 67$ patients and 119 digits, reported an average recurrence and advancement of PIP contracture (39° pre-op and 45° final post-op); however there was 63 % loss to follow-up, possibly indicating successful outcomes in patients who decided no further care was necessary [10]. Overall, minimally invasive partial fasciectomy may result in less maintenance of extension compared with more extensive fasciectomy techniques, but the minimally invasive partial fasciectomy cohorts consistently reported lower rates of complications [10, 15, 16, 21, 23]. At final follow-up, minimally invasive partial fasciectomy has displayed excellent success in the MCP joints treated, while correction of affected PIP joints has resulted in variable rates and degrees of maintained extension [10, 15, 16].

Two nonsurgical techniques have been proposed, and accepted with some popularity in the management of Dupuytren's. Percutaneous needle aponeurectomy sections Dupuytren's cords at various levels. This technique has yielded good early results and patient satisfaction, but long-term results and successes in patients with severe disease have been less than satisfactory [7, 12]. One drawback to this technique is that PNA forgoes the cord visualization afforded by minimally invasive fasciectomy, theoretically increasing the risk of neurovascular injury [10]. Another nonoperative technique, collagenase injections, aims to lyse cords and has been reported to have excellent short-term results with a low side effect profile [8, 11]. However, due to its relative infancy as an intervention option, there is a paucity of long-term data. A single long-term study reports collagenase has high rates of MCP joint recurrence (67 %) and recurrence with increased severity of PIP joint disease as compared to pre-injection measures (45° pre-injection to 60° at final follow-up) [24]. Collagenase also has a high cost assumption, often not covered by insurance plans, and is generally not considered to be a cost-effective therapy [13, 14, 25].

Open fasciectomy and its derivatives, including limited fasciectomy, are commonly used surgical techniques in the management of Dupuytren's. These fasciectomy procedures incorporate a variety of incisional patterns which can be fairly invasive, involving extensive dissection [1, 26–29]. Compared to minimally invasive partial fasciectomy, limited fasciectomy has the advantage of greater visualization of diseased tissue and neurovascular structures; however it may create a greater traumatic inflammatory response from more extensive dermal disruption. Despite lower rates of recurrence and disease extension, the variants of open fasciectomy have been associated with high rates of complications, both intraoperatively and postoperatively [28–30]. Neurovascular injury, infection, flare reaction, and/or hematoma among other complications have been reported in up to 30.8 % those undergoing primary fasciectomy [30].

For the patient in this vignette, an elderly man with a multitude of risk factors and mild-moderate disease of the right fourth digit with PIP involvement, numerous treatment options exist. Due to MCP contracture of >30° and PIP involvement, nonsurgical options were ruled out, per standard practice [1, 8]. The decision to proceed with a minimally invasive technique was made as a result of the patient's advanced age at presentation and relatively limited distribution of the disease. The only reservation in making the choice to proceed with minimally invasive partial fasciectomy was based on PIP involvement of 80°. However, given the patient's age and overall health, the prospective of a quick return to activity with reduced risk of postoperative complication outweighed the potential for disease recurrence or extension. Generally, minimally invasive partial fasciectomy can be considered as a surgical option for patients presenting with mild-moderate disease with limited or no PIP involvement, and the desire for a less invasive surgical option with an expeditious return to daily activities.

Clinical Pearls/Pitfalls

- Patient selection for minimally invasive partial fasciectomy should exclude patients with advanced disease, Dupuytren's diathesis, or significant PIP joint involvement.
- Patient selection should include those with mild-moderate disease, including those with limited PIP involvement, if rapid return to activity or a less invasive surgical procedure is desired.
- Visualization and isolation of neurovascular bundles with reverse Hohmann retractors is both helpful and necessary to avoid iatrogenic neurovascular injuries.
- If safe visualization is not obtained, the cord release must be forgone to judicially protect neurovascular structures.
- Early range of motion is encouraged, as is a period of extension splinting, particularly at night over the initial 4–6 postoperative period.

References

1. Black EM, Blazer PE. Dupuytren disease: an evolving understanding of an age-old disease. J Am Acad Orthop Surg. 2011;19:746–57.
2. Coert JH, Barret JP, Meek MF. Results of partial fasciectomy for Dupuytren disease in 261 consecutive patients. Ann Plast Surg. 2006;57:13–7.
3. Dolmans GH, Werker PM, Hennies HC, et al. Wnt signaling and Dupuytren's disease. N Engl J Med. 2011;365:307–17.
4. Murrell GA, Francis MJ, Howlett CR. Dupuytren's contracture: fine structure in relation to aetiology. J Bone Joint Surg Br. 1989;71(3):367–73.
5. Burke FD, Proud G, Lawson IJ, McGoech KL, Miles JN. An assessment of the effects of exposure to vibration, smoking, alcohol and diabetes on the prevalence of Dupuytren's disease in 97,537 miners. J Hand Surg Eur. 2007;32(4):400–6.
6. Burge P, Hoy G, Regan P, Milne R. Smoking, alcohol and the risk of Dupuytren's contracture. J Bone Joint Surg Br. 1997;79(2):206–10.
7. Pess GM, Pess RM, Pess RA. Results of needle aponeurotomy for Dupuytren contracture in over 1,000 fingers. J Hand Surg Am. 2012; 37A:351–6.
8. Glickel SZ. Update on surgery of the hand. J Am Acad Orthop Surg. 2013;21(4):202–3.
9. Eaton C. Percutaneous fasciotomy for Dupuytren's contracture. J Hand Surg Am. 2011;36:910–5.
10. Gelman S, Schlenker R, Bachoura A, Jacoby SM, Lipman J, Shin EK, Culp RW. Minimally invasive partial fasciectomy for Dupuytren's contractures. Hand. 2012;7:364–9.
11. Srinivasan RC, Shah SH, Jebson PJ. New treatment options for Dupuytren's surgery: collagenase and percutaneous aponeurotomy. J Hand Surg Am. 2010;35:1362–4.
12. Chen NC, Srinivasan RC, Shauver MJ, Chung KC. A systematic review of outcomes of fasciotomy, aponeurotomy, and collagenase treatments for Dupuytren's contracture. Hand. 2011;6:250–5.
13. Baltzer H, Binhammer PA. Cost-effectiveness in the management of Dupuytren's contracture. A Canadian cost-utility analysis of current and future management strategies. Bone Joint J. 2013;95B(8):1094–100.
14. Chen NC, Shauver MJ, Chung KC. Cost-effectiveness of open partial fasciectomy, needle aponeurotomy, and collagenase injection for Dupuytren contracture. J Hand Surg Am. 2011;36A:1826–34.
15. Lee H, Eo S, Cho S, Jones NF. The surgical release of Dupuytren's contracture using multiple transverse incisions. Arch Plast Surg. 2012;39(4):426–30.
16. Shin EK, Jones NF. Minimally invasive technique for release of Dupuytren's contracture: segmental fasciectomy through multiple transverse incisions. Hand. 2011;6:256–9.

17. Tonkin MA, Burke FD, Varian JP. Dupuytren's contracture: a comparative study of fasciectomy and dermatofasciectomy. J Hand Surg Br. 1984;9: 156–62.
18. Chick LR, Lister GD. Surgical alternatives in Dupuytren's contracture. Hand Clin. 1991;7(4):715–9.
19. Becker GW, Davis TRC. The outcome of surgical treatments for primary Dupuytren's disease—a systematic review. J Hand Surg Eur. 2010; 35E(8):623–6.
20. McCash CR. The open palm technique in Dupuytren's contracture. Br J Plast Surg. 1964;17:271–80.
21. Moermans JP. Long-term results after segmental aponeurectomy for Dupuytren's disease. J Hand Surg Br. 1996;21:797–800.
22. Citron N, Hearnden A. Skin tension in the aetiology of Dupuytren's disease: a prospective trial. J Hand Surg Br. 2003;28:528–30.
23. Moermans JP. Segmental aponeurectomy in Dupuytren's disease. J Hand Surg Br. 1991;16:243–54.
24. Watt AJ, Curtin CM, Hentz VR. Collagenase injection as nonsurgical treatment of Dupuytren's disease: 8-year follow-up. J Hand Surg Am. 2010; 35:534–9.
25. Canadian Agency for Drugs and Technologies in Health. Needle or open fasciotomy for Dupuytren's contracture: a review of the comparative efficacy, safety and cost-effectiveness—an update. Rapid response report: summary with critical appraisal. November 11, 2013.
26. Ullah AS, Dias JJ, Bhowal B. Does a 'firebreak' full-thickness skin graft prevent recurrence after surgery for Dupuytren's contracture?: a prospective, randomized trial. J Bone Joint Surg Br. 2009;91:374–8.
27. Freehafer AA, Strong JM. The treatment of Dupuytren's contracture by partial fasciectomy. J Bone Joint Surg. 1963;45A(6):1207–16.
28. Anwar MU, Al Ghazal SK, Boome RS. Results of surgical treatment of Dupuytren's disease in women: a review of 109 consecutive patients. J Hand Surg Am. 2007;32:1423–8.
29. Misra A, Jain A, Ghazanfar R, Johnston T, Nanchahal J. Predicting the outcome of surgery for the proximal interphalangeal joint in Dupuytren's disease. J Hand Surg. 2007;32A:240–5.
30. Denkler K. Surgical complications associated with fasciectomy for Dupuytren's disease: a 20-year review of the English literature. Eplasty. 2010;10:e15.

Suggested Readings

Gelman S, et al. Minimally invasive partial fasciectomy for Dupuytren's contractures. Hand. 2012;7(4):364–9.
Shin EK, Jones NF. Minimally invasive technique for release of Dupuytren's contracture; segmental fasciectomy through multiple transverse incisions. Hand. 2011;6:256–9.

Chapter 7
Surgical Fasciotomy for Dupuytren Contracture

Reid W. Draeger and Peter J. Stern

Case Presentation

A 54-year-old right-handed homemaker presented for evaluation of progressive "drawing in" of the right middle and ring fingers. She began to notice skin puckering in her palm approximately 2 years prior to presentation. She was able to fully straighten the fingers until approximately 6 months prior to presentation at which time the fingers became progressively more contracted and daily activities became more difficult due to loss of finger extension.

R.W. Draeger, MD (✉)
Department of Orthopaedics, School of Medicine, University of North Carolina, Campus Box #7055, 3102 Bioinformatics Building, Chapel Hill, NC 27599-7055, USA
e-mail: reid_draeger@med.unc.edu

P.J. Stern, MD
Department of Orthopaedic Surgery, College of Medicine, University of Cincinnati, 231 Albert Sabin Way, Cincinnati, OH 45207, USA
e-mail: pstern@handsurg.com

© Springer International Publishing Switzerland 2016   83
M. Rizzo (ed.), *Dupuytren's Contracture*,
DOI 10.1007/978-3-319-23841-8_7

On physical examination, tight pretendinous cords were appreciated to the right middle and ring fingers (Fig. 7.1). The contractures were confined to the MCP joints of both digits, with the PIP and DIP joints spared. Range of motion was as follows: right middle finger MCP 30/90°, PIP 0/100°, DIP 0/70°; right ring finger MCP 40/90°, PIP 0/100°, DIP 0/70°. Sensibility was normal and there was brisk capillary refill in all digits. No Garrod nodes or other sites of ectopic disease were present. The patient's family history was unremarkable for Dupuytren contracture.

Diagnosis/Assessment

The diagnosis of Dupuytren contracture, in most cases, is confirmed with history and physical examination. There is no role for laboratory evaluation or advanced imaging. Dupuytren nodules alone may be confused with volar retinacular ganglion cysts or tender A1 pulleys associated with trigger digits. However, palpation of a cord helps to firm up the diagnosis of Dupuytren contracture. Though rare, consideration of palmar fasciitis and contracture secondary to a paraneoplastic syndrome should be considered in all patients, especially female, non-Caucasian patients, in which Dupuytren contracture is uncommon, and in those patients with acutely painful hands, as is associated with polyarthritis and post-traumatic conditions (i.e., distal radius fracture) [1].

Evaluation of all patients with suspected Dupuytren contracture should include questions about family history, ectopic sites of involvement, bilateral involvement, and patient age at original onset. Positive family history, ectopic lesions (Garrod nodes, Peyronie disease, and Ledderhose disease), bilateral hand involvement, original onset before age 50, and male gender are all factors used to determine a diagnosis of Dupuytren diathesis, which portends a much more aggressive course of disease than isolated Dupuytren contracture.

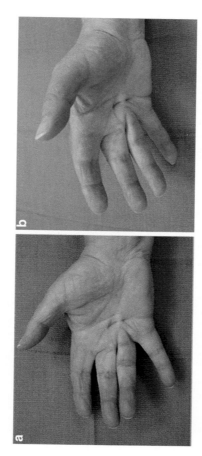

Fig. 7.1 (**a** and **b**) Preoperative view of the patient's hand (**a**: palmar view, **b**: oblique view) (Photographs courtesy of Richard Kang, MD)

Management

The decision of which of the myriad treatments for Dupuytren contracture to pursue is not only dependent on the characteristics of the patient's disease, but also patient preference. We are strong believers in shared decision making with the patient on treatment selection for Dupuytren disease.

In general, we have found limited fasciotomy to be most effective for contractures at the MCP joints. In patients with multiple involved digits or those whose health status precludes a regional or general anesthetic, limited fasciotomy provides a reliable, simple, treatment for the contractures in a single procedure. Limited fasciotomy was chosen to treat this patient's moderate contractures of her long and ring finger MCP joints.

The incision for a limited fasciotomy is transverse and planned directly over the most prominent and taut portion of the pathologic cord or cords. For most MCP contractures, this will be around the level of the distal palmar crease (Fig. 7.2). The skin is incised and the skin is dissected off of the underlying cord. Dissection is carried both radially and ulnarly around the cord to ensure no inter-

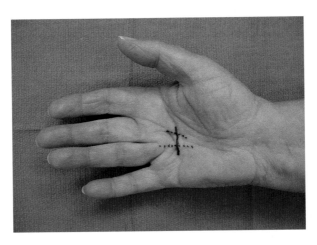

Fig. 7.2 Planned surgical incision (Photograph courtesy of Richard Kang, MD)

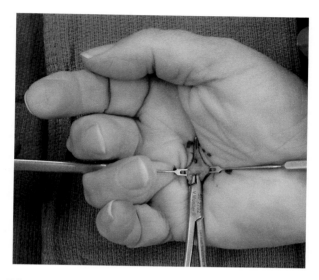

Fig. 7.3 The skin is dissected off of the underlying cord and a hemostat is placed under the cord, carefully isolating it from the surrounding neurovascular structures. The cord to the ring finger is isolated (Photograph courtesy of Richard Kang, MD)

vening neurovascular structures are in danger at the planned fasciotomy site (Figs. 7.3 and 7.4). The isolated cords are then transversely incised leaving the surrounding palmar fascia intact (Fig. 7.5). Once the cord has been divided, the patient is asked to fully extend the fingers to evaluate the success of the fasciotomy (Fig. 7.6). The wound is left open to heal by secondary intention. A sterile soft dressing is applied and the patient is encouraged to flex and extend the fingers immediately postoperatively.

Outcome

The patient underwent limited fasciotomy of her long and ring finger MCP Dupuytren contractures. Immediate postoperative range of motion was initiated and at 5 days, a resting night splint

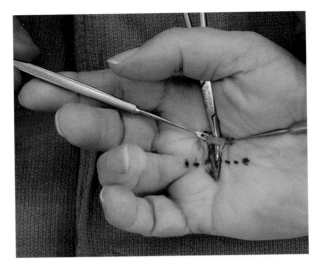

Fig. 7.4 The cord to the long finger has been isolated from surrounding neurovascular structures with a hemostat placed beneath the cord. The cord to the ring finger has been transversely sectioned (Photograph courtesy of Richard Kang, MD)

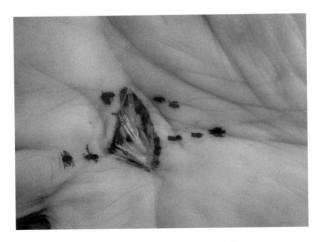

Fig. 7.5 The longitudinal cords to both the long and ring finger have been cut, and surrounding structures, including the nonpathologic fibers of the palmar fascia, are left intact (Photograph courtesy of Richard Kang, MD)

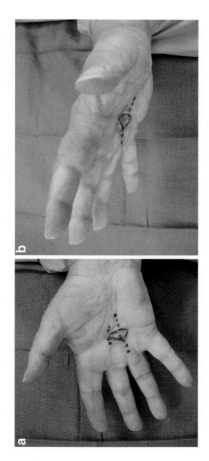

Fig. 7.6 (**a** and **b**) View of the patient's hand with attempted active intraoperative extension shows no residual contracture at the MCP joints of either the long or ring fingers (**a**: palmar view, **b**: lateral view) (Photographs courtesy of Richard Kang, MD)

was fabricated to maintain digital extension. Immediately following fasciotomy, the long and ring fingers were actively extended to 0°. This was maintained through the early postoperative period at 1 week (Fig. 7.7) and 3 weeks (Fig. 7.8). Initially, the patient had difficulty with tight grip activities due to her palmar wound, but this normalized by 3 weeks postoperatively. The patient's wound healed secondarily without complications. After the healing of her palmar wound, the patient was told to follow-up if she noticed recurrence or worsening of the contractures. She has not returned to our clinic for recurrence or worsening of her contractures.

Literature Review

Open fasciotomy for Dupuytren contracture was one of the earliest described treatments for the condition. Both Sir Astley Cooper in 1823 and Dupuytren himself in 1834 described such a treatment and found that it was successful [2, 3]. Fasciotomy requires much less extensive dissection than fasciectomy. Also, because the neurovascular structures can be clearly identified and protected during an open fasciotomy, risk of damage to neurovascular structures is lower than in procedures in which these structures are not visualized, such as percutaneous needle aponeurotomy [4].

Little has been written on open surgical fasciotomy for the treatment of Dupuytren contracture and reports are generally retrospective case series. Patient selection for open fasciotomy is important. Results from multiple series indicate that patients with MCP contractures experienced better results with fasciotomy than patients with contractures at the PIP joint [2, 5]. Rowley et al. found the correction of digits with predominately MCP contractures to be fairly well sustained for an average of 15 month follow-up [2]. However, Bryan and Ghorbal found that these results deteriorated over time and that even amongst those patients with predominately MCP contractures, only 57 % maintained their correction at 5 years postoperatively [5]. Because of this relatively high recurrence rate, these authors recommended

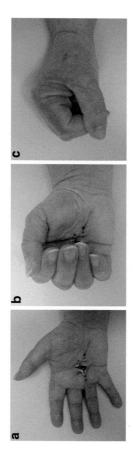

Fig. 7.7 (**a–c**) Views of the patient's hand at 1 week postoperatively. (**a**) Palmar view shows healthy wound bed. (**b**) Palmar clenched fist view and (**c**) lateral clenched fist view show that the patient has some residual stiffness (Photographs courtesy of Richard Kang, MD)

fasciotomy for treatment of unhealthy or elderly patients with contractures predominately at the MCP joint [2, 5].

Some authors have not limited their indications for fasciotomy to contractures of the MCP joint alone. Colville treated contractures of both the MCP joints and the PIP joints with fasciotomy incisions placed as distally at the PIP flexion crease, but reported mixed results with this technique with an average 75° total extensor lag between the MCP and PIP joints by 3 years postoperatively [6]. A more recent report from Stewart, et al. offers more promising results of open fasciotomy. At 5 years follow-up, these authors achieved a "complete release" in 93 % of digits using a transverse incision in the palm for MCP contractures and at the palmodigital crease and PIP crease for PIP contractures [4]. According to this report, 9 % of patients required a revision surgery after undergoing open fasciotomy at an average of 4 years postoperatively. Patients who underwent fasciotomy incisions in both the palm and the digit were more likely to develop more severe recurrent disease than those patients with isolated releases in the palm [4].

Despite wounds being left open to heal by secondary intention in most of these series, reports of complications are minimal, with only one wound complication (treated successfully with oral antibiotics) [4]. Other complications, including neurovascular complications, have been minimal, with reported nerve injuries always being transient [4, 6].

No studies to our knowledge have directly compared contracture correction, recurrence, or complications of open surgical fasciotomy to percutaneous needle aponeurotomy. Though recurrence is often not universally defined, series of percutaneous needle aponeurotomy have shown recurrence rates of around 50 % at 3 years postoperatively [7–9], which is likely comparable or slightly higher than recurrence rates following open fasciotomy [2, 4, 5]. Though nerve lacerations are uncommon with both percutaneous needle aponeurotomy (<1 %) [7–9] and open fasciotomy (0 %) [2, 4, 5], the direct visualization of the Dupuytren cords and the neurovascular bundles in open fasciotomy may help to minimize the risk of nerve-related complications.

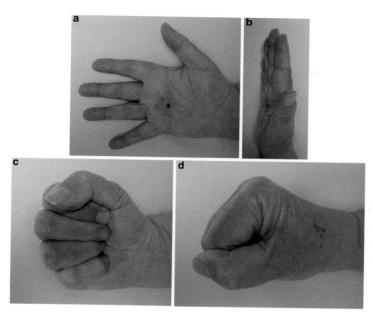

Fig. 7.8 (**a–d**) Views of the patient's hand at 3 weeks postoperatively. (**a**) Palmar view shows the wound nearly healed by secondary intention with no sign of infection. (**b**) Lateral view shows no residual contracture at the long or ring finger MCP joints. (**c**) Palmar clenched fist view and (**d**) lateral clenched fist view show that the patient can easily make a tight composite fist with no residual stiffness (Photographs courtesy of Richard Kang, MD)

Clinical Pearls/Pitfalls

- Fasciotomy is most effective for isolated contractures of the MCP joint.
- A transverse incision is placed over the most prominent/subcutaneous portion of the offending cord(s). This usually is around the area of the distal palmar crease, but do not hesitate to deviate from the crease if another location seems better suited for the fasciotomy.

- Do not hesitate to extend the surgical incision transversely to ensure that the cord can be completely isolated from surrounding neurovascular structures prior to sectioning the cord.
- Leave the wound open to close by secondary intention. This lessens tension on the wound site, which may help minimize recurrence. Local wound care is required initially; however, most patients are able to successfully heal the transverse incision by secondary intention.

Acknowledgement The authors would like to thank Dr. Richard Kang, MD, for use of the photos appearing in this case.

References

1. Manger B, Schett G. Palmar fasciitis and polyarthritis syndrome-systematic literature review of 100 cases. Semin Arthritis Rheum. 2014;44(1):105–11.
2. Rowley DI, Couch M, Chesney RB, Norris SH. Assessment of percutaneous fasciotomy in the management of Dupuytren's contracture. J Hand Surg (Edinburgh, Scotland). 1984;9(2):163–4.
3. Dupuytren G. Permanent retraction of the fingers, produced by an affection of the palmar fascia. Lancet. 1834;2:222–5.
4. Stewart C, Davidson D, Hooper G. Re-operation after open fasciotomy for Dupuytren's disease in a series of 1077 consecutive operations. J Hand Surg Eur Vol. 2013;39(5):553–4.
5. Bryan AS, Ghorbal MS. The long-term results of closed palmar fasciotomy in the management of Dupuytren's contracture. J Hand Surg (Edinburgh, Scotland). 1988;13(3):254–6.
6. Colville J. Dupuytren's contracture—the role of fasciotomy. Hand. 1983;15(2):162–6.
7. Foucher G, Medina J, Navarro R. Percutaneous needle aponeurotomy: complications and results. J Hand Surg (Edinburgh, Scotland). 2003;28(5):427–31.
8. Pess GM, Pess RM, Pess RA. Results of needle aponeurotomy for Dupuytren contracture in over 1,000 fingers. J Hand Surg. 2012;37(4):651–6.
9. van Rijssen AL, Werker PM. Percutaneous needle fasciotomy in Dupuytren's disease. J Hand Surg (Edinburgh, Scotland). 2006;31(5):498–501.

Suggested Readings

Bryan AS, Ghorbal MS. The long-term results of closed palmar fasciotomy in the management of Dupuytren's contracture. J Hand Surg (Edinburgh, Scotland). 1988;13(3):254–6.

Colville J. Dupuytren's contracture—the role of fasciotomy. Hand. 1983;15(2):162–6.

Dupuytren G. Permanent retraction of the fingers, produced by an affection of the palmar fascia. Lancet. 1834;2:222–5.

Rowley DI, Couch M, Chesney RB, Norris SH. Assessment of percutaneous fasciotomy in the management of Dupuytren's contracture. J Hand Surg (Edinburgh, Scotland). 1984;9(2):163–4.

Stewart C, Davidson D, Hooper G. Re-operation after open fasciotomy for Dupuytren's disease in a series of 1077 consecutive operations. J Hand Surg Eur Vol. 2013;39(5):553–4.

Chapter 8
Surgical Fasciectomy for Dupuytren's Contracture

Nathan Douglass and Jeffrey Yao

Case Presentation

A 54-year-old right-hand dominant woman presented to our clinic with recurrent contracture of the ulnar side of her left hand consistent with Dupuytren's disease. A partial surgical fasciectomy involving the small finger had been performed 6 years prior by another surgeon. Postoperatively she participated in hand therapy and nighttime splinting, but her disease gradually returned. Her chief complaint was difficulty with activities of daily living due to her contractures. Examination demonstrated a 10° contracture of the long finger MCP, 20° and 80° contractures of the ring finger MCP and PIP, respectively, and 30° and 30° contractures of the small finger MCP and PIP, respectively.

N. Douglass, MD (✉) • J. Yao, MD
Department of Orthopaedic Surgery, Stanford University Medical Center, 450 Broadway Street, Redwood City, CA 94063, USA
e-mail: ndouglass@gmail.com; jyao@stanford.edu

© Springer International Publishing Switzerland 2016
M. Rizzo (ed.), *Dupuytren's Contracture*,
DOI 10.1007/978-3-319-23841-8_8

Concepts of Surgical Management

Dupuytren's is a chronic disease without a known cure. Although surgical fasciectomy often produces the appearance of a short-term cure without recognizable residual disease, there is a permanent risk of new or recurrent disease. Even with meticulous microdissection of all visible disease, new or recurrent foci of disease may appear in the long term. Unlike a tumor with margins, Dupuytren's disease is an underlying disorder of tissue and therefore "margins" are unclear or nonexistent during surgery. One must also consider the potential for worsening of the inflammatory disease process after surgery. Dupuytren's disease is an abnormal fibroproliferative reaction to tensile forces and surgical management focuses on elimination of diseased tissue and shielding the hand from such tensile forces, including residual skin. Residual mechanical stress across the diseased areas may increase fibroblast proliferation and recurrence of contractures [1–3].

Indications

Surgical treatment of Dupuytren's disease is an elective procedure and usually undertaken once the hand begins to lose function. Contractures of the MCP and PIP joints are most common reasons for surgery, although web space contractures may also interfere with grasp or pinch. The tabletop hand test is an excellent and easy metric for both surgeons and patients to follow clinically [4]. As contractures develop past 30° in the MCP joints or 15–20° in the PCP joints, the hand is unable to be placed flat on a table. This is the typical severity of contracture that leads to the consideration of surgery. Contractures of the first web space between thumb and index finger may affect hand function significantly (Fig. 8.1a–d). Contractures that are borderline for surgical consideration without progression or functional impact are reasonably treated with observation. On the other hand, worsening contractures reliably progress and interfere with functional tasks of daily living.

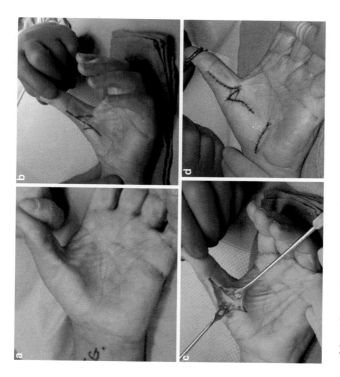

Fig. 8.1 Contracture of the web space between the thumb and index finger is demonstrated preoperatively (**a**). A Z-plasty incision (**b**) was utilized, with a cord identified for excision intraoperatively (**c**) and closure (**d**) with concomitant carpal tunnel release

The decision to pursue treatment must take into consideration the context of the disease including the severity of the disease, patient age and comorbidities, and patient expectations. Evaluation of disease severity includes its rate of progression, degree of contractures, concomitant lower extremity plantar or penile disease, and functional losses. At the same time, patients with mild but worsening contractures should be counseled that the surgery required to correct contractures becomes more complex and the results less predictable as the contractures worsen. As with other joints in the body that are immobilized for long periods of time, the joint capsule, collateral ligaments, and other surrounding tissues of the digits will contribute to contractures over time and may require more aggressive treatment to correct.

Setup

Operative procedures for Dupuytren's disease are best performed with regional peripheral nerve blockade (supra- or infraclavicular block) with light sedation in an ambulatory surgical center. The patient is placed in the supine position with the aid of a hand table. The upper extremity is draped in the usual sterile fashion, and the limb exsanguinated with an Esmarch elastic bandage and inflatable tourniquet. Intravenous antibiotics are given prior to incision. We prefer to use the universal hand holder and retractor set for positioning of hand and digits.

Open Surgical Techniques

Open surgical treatment of Dupuytren's disease is classified as segmental fasciectomy, limited fasciectomy, dermatofasciectomy, or radical fasciectomy.

The once popular radical fasciectomy [5] has largely fallen out of favor owing to its increased morbidity without demonstrable improvement in recurrence rates. In radical fasciectomy, the entire palmar fascia is excised, including fascia that is normal in appearance. In theory radical fasciectomy eliminates active and future sources of disease. However, evidence has demonstrated significant recurrence rates nonetheless [6].

Limited fasciectomy remains the mainstay for open treatment of Dupuytren's disease. Surgery focuses on removal of the bulk of diseased tissue and correction of contractures, with limited dissection otherwise. The goal is to excise enough diseased tissue in order to obtain functional improvements with the understanding that recurrence or disease extension may occur in the long term.

Dermatofasciectomy involves a limited fasciectomy with excision of skin intimately involved with the underlying disease (Fig. 8.2a–d). The defect in the volar digit or palm is filled with full thickness skin grafting. Proponents theorize that the normal skin graft acts as a barrier to disease recurrence, although recurrence still may occur [7, 8]. Surgeons typically utilize dermatofasciectomy more often in cases of greater disease burden, including recurrence or in younger patients with severe disease [7–9].

Moermans [10] described the use of multiple segmental aponeurectomies or fasciectomies through the use of multiple 1–1.5 cm curved incisions, which if joined together would form a lazy "S." The multiple defects create discontinuities in the contractures allowing correction of the contracture with limited removal of diseased tissue.

Incisions

Many skin incisions have been described for fasciotomy or fasciectomy. The incision chosen should allow for adequate exposure without threatening skin flap viability, resection of diseased skin when indicated, and allow tension-free closures after the correction of contractures. In general, longitudinal incisions may be easily extended and provide good intraoperative visualization of primarily longitudinal anatomic structures. Transverse incisions are popular in the palm, including Dupuytren's original description for fasciotomy. The type of incision chosen depends more on the foci

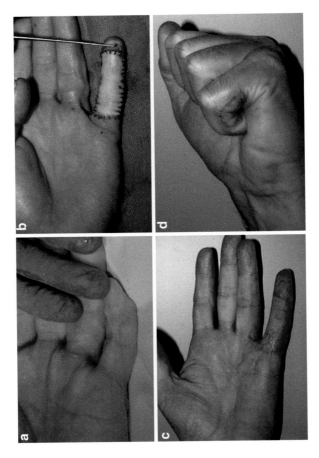

Fig. 8.2 Contractures affecting the small finger PIP and DIP joint preoperatively (**a**) were treated with dermatofasciectomy and skin grafting (**b**). Postoperative images demonstrating appearance and range of motion (**c, d**)

of disease and surgeon preference than the superiority of any particular incision type. Often, multiple incisions and combinations of types are used in a single procedure. For revision surgery, as was the case with the patient presented here, previous incisions are best utilized and extended as needed.

Longitudinal incisions including Bruner-type zigzag, V-Y advancement, Z-plasty (Fig. 8.3a–d), and midaxial (Fig. 8.4a, b) incisions are well suited for exposure of the longitudinal anatomical structures of the hand and digits including contracted cords. One randomized study found no difference in recurrence rates amongst two types of longitudinal incisions [11].

In 1964, McCash [12] popularized the open palm technique (Fig. 8.5a–d). McCash made incisions in the transverse palmar creases similar to Dupuytren's original technique. Unlike Dupuytren who incised diseased contractures, McCash performed limited fasciectomies. Upon correction of the contracture and extension of the digits, the resulting skin deficit in the distal palmar crease is left open to heal by secondary intention and treated with a compressive tulle gras dressing and plaster splint. Tulle gras consists of gauze or other weaved fabric impregnated with soft paraffin, or paraffin equivalent. It may also be impregnated with antiseptics or antibiotics. One layer of tulle gras is applied to the open wound followed by a polyvinyl sponge or dry gauze. Firm pressure is applied to the entire hand while a volar plaster slab is placed over the soft dressing with continued pressure until the plaster sets [12].

Longitudinal incisions in the fingers can be combined with open palm technique for the so-called open palm closed fingers technique (Fig. 8.6a–c).

Dissection

Generally the incision begins proximally and proceeds distally. The proximal extent of the incision is determined by the proximal extent of the diseased cord or a natural landmark such as Kaplan's cardinal line. As the diseased pretendinous cord is released proximally, its

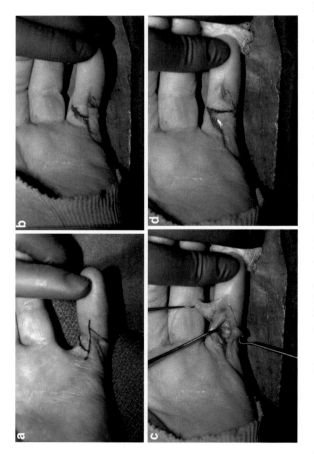

Fig. 8.3 Small finger contracture (**a**) treated with Z-plasty incision (**b**), after cord excision (**c**) and resultant closure (**d**)

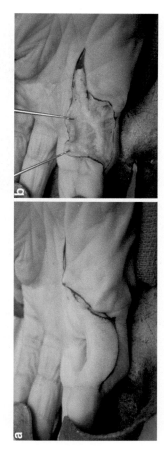

Fig. 8.4 A midaxial incision (**a**) used to treat a small finger PIP contracture from pretendinous and abductor digiti minimi cords (**b**)

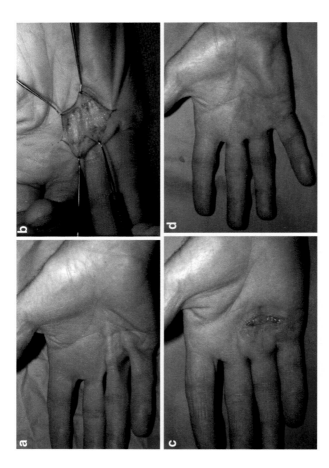

Fig. 8.5 Preoperative clinical photograph (**a**) demonstrating fourth and fifth finger contracture from pretendinous cords seen intraoperatively (**b**). The open palm technique leaves the incision open (**c**). Postoperatively the wound is treated with tulle gras compressive dressing and volar plaster splinting with fingers extended. The wound heals by secondary intention (**d**)

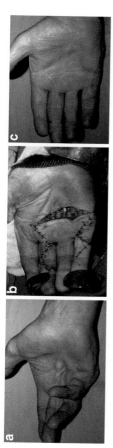

Fig. 8.6 Extensive disease affecting the ulnar three digits (**a**) was treated with the open palm closed finger technique. At the end of the procedure the longitudinal digital incisions were closed and the palmar incision left open (**b**). Subsequent follow-up demonstrates wound healing (**c**)

effect on the distal joints may change and allow easier planning of the distal incisions. There is always concern for injury to the neurovascular bundles. It is helpful to begin the dissection in normal tissue in order to aid in its dissection and for identification and subsequent protection of the neurovascular bundles during mobilization of diseased tissue.

The preoperative exam provides pertinent information about which pathologic cords to expect upon the surgical exposure and minimize risk of neurovascular injury. The common cords resected include the pretendinous, central, spiral, lateral, natatory, abductor digiti minimi, retrovascular, commissural, and radial thumb cord.

Spiral cords present a particular threat and potential for neurovascular injury, particularly with the initial skin incision, as the neurovascular bundle may lie directly underneath the skin on top of the fascia. The spiral cord, originating from four components (pretendinous band, spiral band, lateral digital sheet, and Grayson's ligament), displaces the neurovascular bundle centrally, superficially, and proximally. Surgeons should be suspicious of spiral cords when clinical exam demonstrates a PIP joint contracture with a palpable interdigital soft tissue mass.

PIP Joint Contracture

Resection of diseased tissue and cords reliably corrects MCP contractures yet PIP joint contractures continue to be difficult to correct completely and permanently. Often a PIP contracture may improve but not fully resolve with release of the pathologic cords. Longstanding severe joint contractures potentially affect the joint capsule, volar plate, collateral ligaments, tendons, and surrounding soft tissues.

Severe contractures more reliably achieve a significant degree of improvement whereas less severe contractures, particularly those less than 30°, perform more unpredictably in the long term [13]. If there is residual contracture following standard fasciectomies, tenolysis and tenotomies at varying levels have been advocated [14]. Capsulectomy, volar plate release, and checkrein ligament release have also been proposed [15]. However in one study there was no significant benefit from capsuloligamentous release in addition to fasciectomy alone for severe PIP contractures [16]. Residual PIP contractures of 30° or less after fasciectomy are best left alone without further dissection or release.

Closure

At the end of the procedure the tourniquet is released and great attention is directed towards achieving hemostasis. The vascularity of all digits must be confirmed prior to closure. Vasospasm may be treated first with warm sponges at the time of tourniquet deflation, and then continuous warm irrigation as needed. Finger flexion and local application of smooth muscle relaxants such as lidocaine may be helpful subsequently. If the digit is still not perfusing, the digital arteries should be explored for unrecognized lacerations or rupture. Avascular skin flaps may be trimmed.

Reexamining the neurovascular bundles prior to closure allows immediate repair of unrecognized nerve injuries and eliminates the potential confusion for neuropraxia in the setting of postoperative numbness.

Postoperative hematoma will threaten the viability of overlying skin and provide a nidus for infection, particularly if skin grafts are used. Per surgeon preference, a drain may be placed in the palm and removed the next day in the office as most procedures now are performed on an outpatient basis.

Skin closure is performed by direct re-approximation, V-Y or Z-plasty, skin grafting, or left open (open palm technique). We prefer closure with interrupted 4-0 nylon sutures, and placement of a compressive dressing followed by plaster splinting with extension at MCP, PIP, and DIP joints. Tulle gras is a popular material for wound bandaging and consists of a weave fabric impregnated with soft paraffin placed directly onto the closed or open wound.

Follow-Up

The patient follows up in clinic 1 week postoperatively for splint removal and assessment of the incisions. Hand therapy is begun at that point with aggressive flexion/extension of the digits. The hand therapist fashions an MCP/PIP/DIP joint extension splint for nighttime use only. The patient returns 2 weeks postoperatively for reassessment of wounds and suture removal. The patient is instructed in wound care and scar massage.

When performing the open palm technique, the patient begins opening and closing the hand at 48 h, and the dressing is changed 1 week postoperatively.

Skin grafts require longer immobilization for the graft to take, and are checked beginning postoperative day 2 for hematoma.

Literature Review

Outcomes of Fasciectomy

Reviewing the literature demonstrates difficulties comparing studies given varying definitions of recurrence and follow-up periods. Typically reported recurrence rates range from 8 to 54 % [17] and up to 74 % in the long term [18]. The majority of recurrences occur in the first few years after surgery [19, 20]. In the long term nearly all patients should expect some form of recurrence or extension of disease [17, 21].

Some authors advocate dermatofasciectomy over partial fasciectomy for severe disease with skin involvement or recurrent disease. In some studies dermatofasciectomy has shown lower rates of recurrence and similar rates of extension compared to partial fasciectomy alone [22, 23]. A randomized trial showed no benefit compared to partial fasciectomy and skin closure with Z-plasty, with recurrence rates of 12.2 % at 3 years in both groups [7]. Risk factors for recurrence include young age, knuckle pads, and small finger involvement [19].

Complications

Complications after surgical treatment are expected in 15–20% of patients, but complications causing permanent harm or disability are rare [1]. Surgeons should monitor for hematoma, neurovascular injury, infection, wound necrosis, skin graft failure, stiffness, and postoperative flare or complex regional pain syndrome. Prompt recognition and treatment of complications, particularly neurovascular injuries, will diminish their short- and long-term impacts [24]. Revision surgery and extensive disease increase the difficulty of surgery and likelihood of complication.

Case Presentation

In our patient's procedure, the previous Bruner incision in the small finger was utilized and extended all the way to Kaplan's cardinal line (Fig. 8.7a–d). The pretendinous cord was released proximally and as the cord was brought more distally, the neurovascular bundles were protected. An abductor digiti minimi cord and spiral cord were identified and carefully excised. The MCP and PIP joint of the small finger achieved full extension.

In the ring finger a pretendinous cord was identified. A Bruner incision was used, taking great care to avoid narrow skin flaps. At this point, the cord was identified proximally and released again protecting the neurovascular bundles. Again a spiral cord was identified and complete excision of the Dupuytren's fascia achieved correction of the PIP and MCP joint contractures.

Lastly, the incision from the ring finger was extended over to the long finger and a pretendinous cord was identified and excised correcting the MCP joint contracture.

At 4-year follow-up the patient was found to have full active extension of all joints with the exception of the small finger PIP, which demonstrated a 20° active and 11° passive flexion contracture (Fig. 8.8a–c).

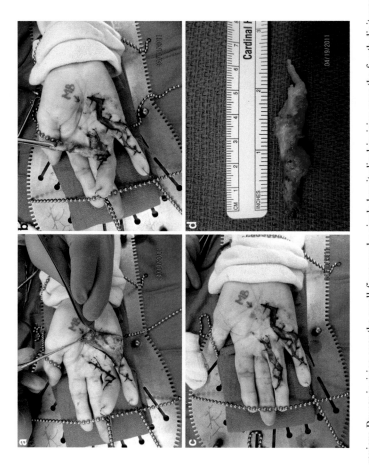

Fig. 8.7 The previous Bruner incision over the small finger and a single longitudinal incision over the fourth digit were utilized and diseased tissue excised (**a**, **b**). Full extension of the digits was achieved (**c**). A typical specimen of excised tissue (**d**)

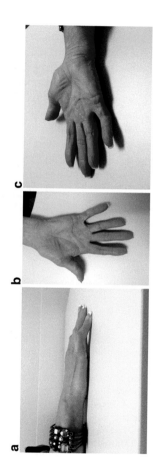

Fig. 8.8 Clinical photographs at 4-year follow-up demonstrate continued improvement of contractures with mild recurrence of the small finger PIP joint contracture (**a**–**c**)

Summary

Dupuytren's disease is a common hand pathology seen in hand and upper extremity clinics. Surgical intervention should be considered when functional disability results from joint or web space contractures. Informed consent must include discussion of the considerable risks of recurrence and extension, based on patient-specific risk factors. Surgery intends to remove clearly diseased tissue with limited dissection into normal tissues. A number of skin incisions and techniques including dermatofasciectomy, skin grafting, and the open palm technique have been described. Each technique or incision has its pros and cons without one being clearly superior in all cases. Vigilant practitioners identify and treat neurovascular injuries and wound complications promptly. Postoperative care focuses on wound healing and early motion. Even in cases of severe and recurrent contractures, surgical fasciectomy for Dupuytren's disease can preserve considerable hand function from an otherwise debilitating condition.

References

1. Eaton C, Seegenschmiedt H, Bayat A, Gabbiani G, Werker P, Wach W. Dupuytren's disease and related hyperproliferative disorders: principles, research, and clinical perspectives. New York, NY: Springer; 2012.
2. McGrouther DA. The microanatomy of Dupuytren's contracture. Hand. 1982;14:215–36.
3. Citron N, Hearnden A. Skin tension in the aetiology of Dupuytren's disease: a prospective trial. J Hand Surg Am. 2003;28B(6):528–30.
4. Hueston JT. The table top test. Hand. 1982;14:100–3.
5. McIndoe A, Beare RL. The surgical management of Dupuytren's contracture. Am J Surg. 1958;95:197–203.
6. Dickie WR, Hughes NC. Dupuytren's contracture: a review of the late results of radical fasciectomy. Br J Plast Surg. 1967;20(1958):311–4.
7. Ullah AS, Dias JJ, Bhowal B. Does a "firebreak" full-thickness skin graft prevent recurrence after surgery for Dupuytren's contracture? A prospective, randomised trial. J Bone Joint Surg Br. 2009;91:374–8.
8. Armstrong JR, Hurren JS, Logan AM. Dermofasciectomy in the management of Dupuytren's disease. J Bone Joint Surg Br. 2000;82:90–4.

9. Black EM, Blazar PE. Dupuytren disease: an evolving understanding of an age-old disease. J Am Acad Orthop Surg. 2011;19:746–57.
10. Moermans JP. Segmental aponeurectomy in Dupuytren's disease. J Hand Surg Br. 1991;16:243–54.
11. Citron ND, Nunez V. Recurrence after surgery for Dupuytren's disease: a randomized trial of two skin incisions. J Hand Surg Am. 2005; 30(6):563–6.
12. McCash CR. The open palm technique in Dupuytren's contracture. Br J Plast Surg. 1964;17:271–80.
13. Legge JW, McFarlane RM. Prediction of results of treatment of Dupuytren's disease. J Hand Surg Am. 1980;5:608–16.
14. Hueston JT. The extensor apparatus in Dupuytren's disease. Ann Chir Main. 1985;4:7–10.
15. Crowley B, Tonkin MA. The proximal interphalangeal joint in Dupuytren's disease. Hand Clin. 1999;15:137–47. viii.
16. Weinzweig N, Culver JE, Fleegler EJ. Severe contractures of the proximal interphalangeal joint in Dupuytren's disease: combined fasciectomy with capsuloligamentous release versus fasciectomy alone. Plast Reconstr Surg. 1996;97(3):560–7.
17. Hurst L. Dupuytren's contracture. In: Hotchkiss RN, Pederson WC, Kozin SH, Wolfe SW, editors. Green's operative hand surgery. 6th ed. Philadelphia: Churchill Livingstone; 2011. p. 141–58.
18. Vigroux JP, Valentin P. A natural history of Dupuytren's contracture treated by surgical fasciectomy: the influence of diathesis (76 hands reviewed at more than 10 years). Ann Chir Main Memb Super. 1992;11:367–74.
19. Hueston JT. Recurrent Dupuytren's contracture. Plast Reconstr Surg. 1963;31(1):66–9.
20. Rebelo JS, Ferreira JB, Vilão MC, Boléo-Tomé J. Dupuytren's disease. Analysis of a 10 year caseload. Acta Med Port. 1992;5:463–6.
21. Hueston JT. Limited fasciectomy for Dupuytren's contracture. Plast Reconstr Surg Transplant Bull. 1961;27(6):569–85.
22. Tonkin MA, Burke FD, Varian JP. Dupuytren's contracture: a comparative study of fasciectomy and dermofasciectomy in one hundred patients. J Hand Surg Br. 1984;9(2):156–62.
23. Ketchum LD, Hixson FP. Dermofasciectomy and full-thickness grafts in the treatment of Dupuytren's contracture. J Hand Surg Am. 1987;12:659–64.
24. Boyer MI, Gelberman RH. Complications of the operative treatment of Dupuytren's disease. Hand Clin. 1999;15:161–6. viii.

Chapter 9
Wide Awake Dupuytren's Fasciectomy: A Pathoanatomical Approach

Quamar M.K. Bismil and M.S.K. Bismil

Declarations MSK Bismil and QMK Bismil are founder members of the Worldwide Awake Hand Surgery group and the founders of one-stop wide awake hand surgery.

The Worldwide Awake Hand Surgery Group The Worldwide Awake Hand Surgery group was founded by TH Robbins, MSK Bismil and QMK Bismil circa 2012 and is delighted to assist hand surgeons in their transition to wide awake hand surgery.
www.worldwideawake.net

Q.M.K. Bismil, MBChB, MRCS DipSEM MFSEM DMSMed FRCSEd (✉)
M.S.K. Bismil, MBBS, MS, FRCSEd, DLM
The World Wide Awake Hand Surgery Group, Queen Anne Street
Medical Centre, London W1G 8HU, UK
e-mail: qbismil@gmail.com

© Springer International Publishing Switzerland 2016   117
M. Rizzo (ed.), *Dupuytren's Contracture*,
DOI 10.1007/978-3-319-23841-8_9

One-Stop Wide Awake Dupuytren's Fasciectomy

A 40-year-old man presented to the Wide Awake Hand Surgery clinic with a 15-year history of recurrent deformity of the right dominant ring and little fingers secondary to Dupuytren's contracture. He had previously undergone two operations on the right hand and ring finger elsewhere: these were both conventional fasciectomies performed under general anaesthesia and with a tourniquet. He reported that he had never had a 'straight' ring finger post-surgery. The patient's initial request to the treating surgeons (M.S.K.B. and Q.M.K.B.) was for amputation of both fingers. The patient was fit and well with no history of allergy, took no regular medications and had no history of recreational drug use.

On examination, there was Tubiana stage IV Dupuytren's contracture (Table 9.1) of the ring and little fingers with profound scarring from the previous surgery. There was a fixed proximal interphalangeal (PIP) contracture of the ring finger. There were mobile metacarpophalangeal contractures of both fingers and a mobile PIP contracture of the little finger. Clinically, the ring finger pathoanatomy comprised ulnar-sided central, pretendinous and lateral cords, Grayson's ligament and a natatory cord traversing to the little finger (Fig. 9.1). The central and pretendinous cords were associated with nodular disease. There was no palpable disease in the little finger ray per se. At informed consent, the full range of treatment options, including no treatment and deferred treatment, were discussed. The main treatment options presented were wide awake fasciectomy (either as a one-stop procedure or deferred) and dermofasciectomy (with potential onward referral to a general/regional anaesthesia hand surgeon). The patient was eager to proceed with ring finger wide awake fasciectomy in one management stop [one-stop wide awake (OSWA) fasciectomy].

Table 9.1 Tubiana stages

Tubiana stage	Total degree of contracture (MCP + PIP)
I	Less than 45°
II	Greater than 45°
III	Greater than 90°
IV	Greater than 135°

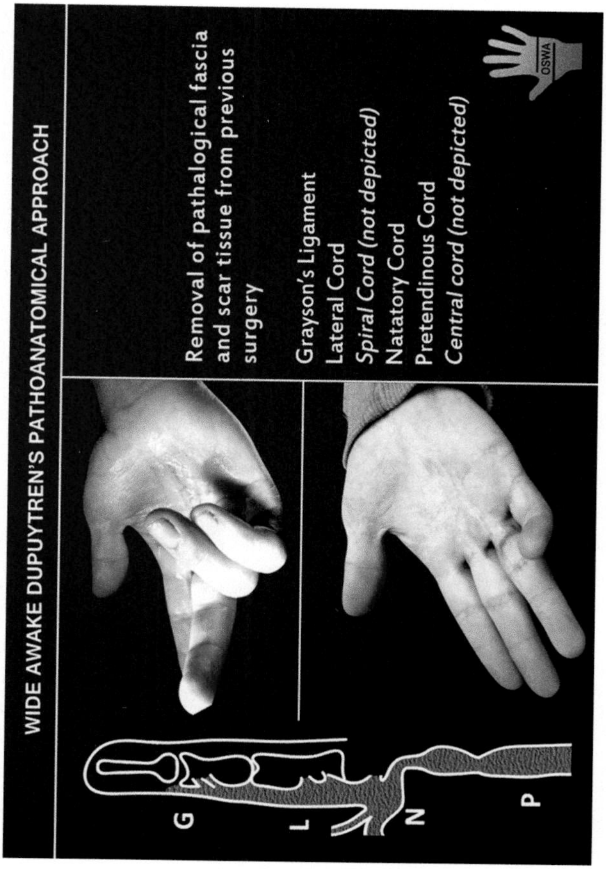

Fig. 9.1 One-stop wide awake Dupuytren's fasciectomy pathoanatomical approach

Wide awake minimally invasive anaesthesia (see appendix, below) for wide awake fasciectomy typically utilises lignocaine 2 % with low-dose adrenaline 1:200,000; the latter acts as a vasopressor and offsets vasodilation from the local anaesthetic. In this case we used 5 ml of lignocaine 2 % with low-dose adrenaline 1:200,000 infiltrated through a 23-gauge needle into the web spaces to anaesthetise the palmar skin. For digits, we prefer plain lignocaine 2 %, infiltrated through the anaesthetised palmar skin using a 21-gauge needle into the volar compartment of the finger at the proximal phalangeal level (in this case, an additional 5 ml of plain lignocaine was used). Smaller needles, say 25–30 gauge, may also be used to minimise injection pain, but in our experience there is a tendency to 'force' the anaesthesia through the smaller needles, especially if there is increased resistance due to the thickened fascia. It should also be noted, as an alternative, that Lalonde and colleagues [1, 2] routinely use lignocaine with low-dose adrenaline for digits as well as for the palm. A key point for all wide awake anaesthesia techniques is that only small pain fibres are blocked and that peripheral nerves are not targeted. Thus, surgery is performed on a moving, sensate hand. In Dupuytren's surgery this means that the flexor tendon mechanism can be assessed dynamically during the procedure, exercises can be demonstrated and understood with full anatomical visualisation during the procedure and the mode of wound closure can be optimised to ensure an ideal (usually full) range of motion is facilitated. The patient is also advised to tell the surgeon immediately if he feels any nerve pain (*tingling/numbness/electric shocks*) as this may help the surgeon when dissecting around the digital nerves. In our experience, the best ways to minimise injection pain include injecting very slowly, using a smaller gauge needle initially to anaesthetise through the web space, advancing the needle tip sequentially through the anaesthetised field and using no larger than a 5-ml syringe to inject (larger syringes may encourage a more vigorous injection technique, in terms of rate and pressure applied). Other options during wide awake anaesthesia include buffering the local anaesthetic (i.e., alkalising it to a more physiological pH) and using a tumescent technique with diluted anaesthetic solution. In our own practice, the former has not been required and the latter is not used routinely in Dupuytren's cases because we do not feel it is particularly helpful for wide awake fasciectomy, where we wish to minimise distortion of the anatomy, especially in relation to the neurovascular bundles. Simple additional methods to minimise injection pain include distraction (through either conversation or audiovisual materials), skin sensory stimulation through gentle 'pinching', meditation/mindfulness techniques and the use of a bone vibrator or similar device on the nearby soft tissues whilst the injections are being delivered. In our experience, all but the most needle-phobic patients are 'happy' to endure usually no more than 30 s of superficial injections for the comfort of tourniquet-free surgery.

In wide awake fasciectomy surgery, as with any fasciectomy technique, anatomical dissection is key: not only enabling visualisation and removal of all macroscopically abnormal fascia, but also obviating the need for a tourniquet. Whereas in conventional fasciectomy the surgeon has the luxury of the tourniquet and a bloodless field, the wide awake hand surgeon must learn to manage bleeding effectively. However, as with conventional fasciectomy, it is principally anatomical dissection and a complete understanding of the pathoanatomy that facilitate an optimal procedure and, in particular, avoidance of any trauma to the palmar arch, digital vessels or their main branches and tributaries. Providing there is no trauma to the larger (i.e., macroscopically visible) palmar or digital vessels, bleeding merely needs to be managed by the wide awake hand surgeon whilst the microvascular bleeding is controlled by primary haemostasis. That is, the wide awake hand surgeon must learn to manage bleeding, especially early in the procedure, whilst awaiting the progression of microvascular constriction and platelet plug formation. This leads to the wide awake hand surgeons' philosophy of bleeding management as 'pressure and time' (see the section entitled 'Discussion'). Thus, through meticulous dissection, point pressure from a rolled swab and primary haemostasis, hand surgeons ensure that as the wide awake fasciectomy proceeds, bleeding becomes progressively less of an issue (as the coagulation cascade progresses and the low-dose adrenaline augments vasoconstriction).

During the wide awake fasciectomy, the diseased cords related to the ring finger were fully removed using the standard technique [3]. In this case, this involved sequential visualisation and fasciectomy of the ulnar-sided pathoanatomy (i.e., central, pretendinous, spiral and lateral cords, Grayson's ligament and the natatory cord traversing to the ring finger). The neurovascular bundles were visualised in their entirety and were heavily involved with scar tissue and also a spiral cord. The flexor mechanism was also encased in scar tissue and was sequentially removed. This necessitated windowing of the flexor sheath, which could be fine-tuned dynamically with active movement. The patient was also asked to move the digit intermittently to enable the surgeon to delineate scar tissue from flexor mechanism.

Extensive skin involvement meant that primary Z-plasty was not feasible since the skin flaps would have been too thin. For the fixed PIP contracture, we performed volar joint capsulotomy, released the checkrein ligaments and released accessory collateral ligaments. During the informed-consent procedure, the standard discussion about deferred Z-plasty (as required) had been included. In fact, in this case deferred Z-plasty was not necessary (see the following section, 'Discussion'). Pre- versus post-operative photographs demonstrate full correction of the ring finger deformity and a good correction of the little finger without any separate surgery having been performed on this ray. The patient was followed up for several months, and there was a significant improvement in all outcome measures.

Discussion: Literature Review

There have been recent developments in the management of Dupuytren's contracture. Ultimately, it is likely that basic science research into the faulty signalling pathways that result in the abnormalities of the palmar fascia in Dupuytren's contracture—and targeting the myofibroblast—will result in a *cure* for the condition later this century. Until then, advances in wide awake hand surgery are likely to play a role in the management of this challenging condition. Broadly, the wide awake treatment options for the management of Dupuytren's contracture causing functional problems are *fasciotomy* (disrupt the diseased tissue with a blind procedure) or *fasciectomy* (remove the diseased tissue with an open procedure). Prior to the advent of wide awake hand surgery, fasciectomy required tourniquets and general/regional anaesthesia/sedation. The avoidance of rare but potentially catastrophic complications of general anaesthesia in the Dupuytren's surgical cohort of often elderly patients is clearly advantageous.

This complex case demonstrates the role of wide awake fasciectomy, with visualisation and removal of the diseased fascia in the wide awake patient, in complex cases. The scarring from previous surgery and the complex disease meant that a blind fasciotomy technique was not appropriate. At informed consent, the patient clearly wished to avoid (the risks of) general anaesthesia, regional anaesthesia, sedation and tourniquets and hence was a good candidate for wide-awake fasciectomy. We invariably adopt a staged approach to Dupuytren's contracture, with each digit assessed and treated separately. Indeed, this case demonstrates that just because multiple digits are affected does not mean that multiple rays require surgery.

Careful consideration of the pathoanatomy enables logical management of Dupuytren's contracture through wide awake fasciectomy. The cause of the little finger involvement in this case was the *natatory cord,* and this was evident from the pre-operative examination. There was no palpable disease in the little finger, but it is likely that the natatory cord that was removed connected to some occult lateral cord disease in the little finger. It is possible that further surgery to the little finger would improve the residual PIP contracture; but without palpable disease in this finger, we elected with the patient to adopt a watchful waiting approach to this digit.

The origins of wide awake Dupuytren's surgery can be traced back to 1981 with TH Robbin's paper [4] on deferred Dupuytren's Z-plasty under local anaesthesia. The rationale for using straight incisions in wide awake Dupuytren's surgery is related to the principles of wide awake hand surgery without tourniquet, as follows. Whilst the use of low-dose adrenaline minimises bleeding (in addition to prolonging the duration of anaesthesia), it does not provide a bloodless field in tourniquet-free wide awake hand surgery. With the advent of wide awake techniques, the risk of tourniquet complications (including swelling, muscular weakness, neurapraxia, hematoma and infection, vascular trauma, necrosis, compartment syndrome and systemic complications) [5] can be avoided. Moreover, there is a limit to the duration of tourniquet use, in terms of pain and the onset of complications. It has been documented that there is finite amount of tourniquet time that an awake hand surgery patient can withstand from a physiological perspective [6].

Straight incisions with or without Z-plasty [4] or Brunner incisions [2, 7] may be used for fasciectomy. However, we primarily utilise straight incisions [3] because bleeding is invariably at its peak at the beginning of the procedure when the incision is being made, so we prefer to use a technique which initially avoids the neurovascular bundle. The wide awake hand surgeons' philosophy of the management of bleeding, 'pressure and time', hinges upon meticulous dissection to avoid any trauma to the vascular macro-anatomy; primary haemostasis; point pressure by the surgeon to control any microvascular bleeding whilst the vessels are constricting and the platelet plug is forming; and promoting vasoconstriction with low-dose adrenaline.

We do not use any form of diathermy for wide awake hand surgery, which underlines the efficacy of the 'pressure and time' philosophy, providing the macrovascular integrity is maintained by the surgeon. By the end of the procedure, the wound should be quite dry, with only minimal ooze from the skin edge and subcutaneous microvasculature. If this is not the case, then the vascular tree in the operative zone should be carefully inspected and any disruption must be dealt with. The logic of wide awake hand surgery in the context of the management of surgical bleeding in fasciectomy is threefold: firstly, it hinges upon a meticulous fasciectomy technique; secondly, rather than preventing bleeding with a tourniquet, the wide awake hand surgeon surgeon respects the coagulation cascade and augments it with the alpha adrenergic effects of low-dose adrenaline on vascular smooth muscle; and thirdly, the wide awake hand surgeon can confidently close the quite dry wound at the end of the procedure, knowing that the vascular tree has not been compromised. Thus, the rather counterintuitive exercise of eliminating all bleeding/blood flow with a tourniquet for the body of the surgical procedure but then deflating the tourniquet prior to closing the wound in order to finally see and manage the bleeding, almost as an afterthought, can now be avoided. By managing the bleeding in a logical, stepwise fashion (Fig. 9.2), the wide awake hand surgeon can confidently close the quite dry wound, knowing that the coagulation cascade will continue to control bleeding, especially if augmented with the modified boxing glove dressing we have described in another publication [3]. We find that inspecting and working around a 'normal' albeit vasoconstricted vascular tree (with the propensity to bleed) during the entire procedure invariably facilitates and ensures the meticulous dissection and preservation of the vascular anatomy that fasciectomy requires. And rather than a race against the tourniquet, the procedure can be conducted at leisure. Moreover, tourniquet-free hand surgery under local anaesthesia empowers the patient to understand his condition and treatment and to take control of his rehabilitation from the point of surgery.

In wide awake hand surgery, bleeding is maximal within the first 5–10 minutes of the procedure given that the onset of the optimal vasoconstrictive effect from epinephrine is around 5 minutes [8] and the bleeding time is invariably less than 10 minutes. This means that the wide awake hand surgeon can reliably predict and manage the bleeding as the procedure progresses. Moreover, in terms of incisions and closure, it is inevitable that by the end of the procedure—provided that meticulous dissection has respected the anatomy—Z-plasties can be sited with the neurovascular bundles under direct vision and without any compromise to vision from bleeding, but the patient has a physiologically 'normal' vascular tree with the propensity to bleed if traumatised. We also prefer Z-plasties as necessary over Brunner incisions because of the 30 % lengthening Z-plasties invariably enable us to achieve. Robbins [4] deferred his Z-plasties as a second procedure as required; this approach was indeed utilised in the case described in this chapter. Ultimately, however, this case did not require a deferred Z-plasty since the scar did not contract and the correction of the deformity was maintained: this is a lesson in itself. Finally, on the subject of incisions and closure, and with regards to our own practice, we should make it clear that our routine method of incision is longitudinal and our routine method of closure is Z-plasty. However, on a case-by-case basis we

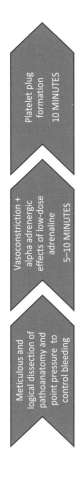

Fig. 9.2 The wide awake hand surgeon's 'pressure and time' approach to bleeding

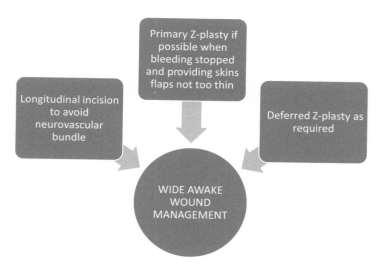

Fig. 9.3 Wide awake wound management within our practice

apply an algorithm as outlined throughout this chapter and as depicted in Fig. 9.3.

Whilst the alpha adrenergic vasoconstrictor effect of low-dose adrenaline is helpful in wide awake fasciectomy for bleeding management and prolongation of the anaesthesia, it is not essential. We have performed many fasciectomies using only plain local anaesthesia and without a vasopressor; invariably, meticulous dissection, management of ooze with point pressure and the patient's coagulation cascade facilitate a technically successful wide awake fasciectomy without bleeding complication. Patients with coagulopathy or bleeding diathesis should be carefully evaluated in conjunction with their haematologist before any treatment is offered for their Dupuytren's condition. If any contraindications to low-dose adrenaline/vasopressor exist, use plain local anaesthesia. As surgeons plan their transition to wide awake hand surgery, they should carefully select their patients. The use of plain local anaesthesia should be reserved only for the more experienced wide awake hand surgeon since such procedures are inevitably more challenging.

With wide awake fasciectomy, the patient is involved in an immediate patient-centred rehabilitative approach with the pathology, surgery and rehabilitation demonstrated on table and with full visualisation of the (patho-)anatomy. With the wide awake approach, the patient is shown her post-operative exercises on the table and accelerated rehabilitation commences immediately (range-of-motion exercises, mid-range). Further active movement (full, including end-range) commences according to comfort as soon as the modified boxing glove bandage is removed (i.e., after 1 week). The modified boxing glove bandage [3] has been used by the senior author (MSKB) for several decades; along with the 'pressure and time' approach to the management of bleeding in hand surgery, it has eliminated significant post-operative haematoma in Dupuytren's fasciectomy patients [3]. Thus, we have not had any returns to theatre for bleeding or infection since the foundation of the Wide Awake Hand Surgery service here in the United Kingdom in 1999. Passive daily stretching commences once the wound is healed. For patients such as the gentleman described here who opt for a one-stop pathway, the rehabilitation taught during the procedure is supplemented with web video. Also, patients have uninterrupted access to the surgeon via a telephone helpline and email. Scar massage and scar desensitisation techniques are taught as required, often remotely using web resources (see Fig. 9.4).

The patient's perception and approach to the benefits versus risks of management options are key in logical decision making during the informed-consent process (Fig. 9.5). Other than wide awake fasciectomy, options include fasciotomy with a needle or an enzymatic injection and dermofasciectomy under general or regional anaesthetic.

We are reluctant to perform blind fasciotomy techniques in complex disease configurations or revision cases since the proximity of the digital nerves and tendons jeopardises these structures when 'normal' anatomy is distorted. For a simple pretendinous or central cord, a fasciotomy procedure would always be offered at informed consent as an alternative to wide awake fasciectomy. Now that Dupuytren's fasciectomy with accelerated rehabilitation can routinely be performed wide awake [1, 9, 10], it is our experience that the majority of patients, like the patient presently discussed, would not wish to consider dermofasciectomy under

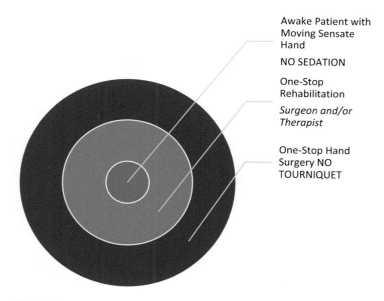

Awake Patient with
Moving Sensate
Hand

NO SEDATION

One-Stop
Rehabilitation

*Surgeon and/or
Therapist*

One-Stop Hand
Surgery NO
TOURNIQUET

Fig. 9.4 One-stop wide awake Dupuytren's fasciectomy

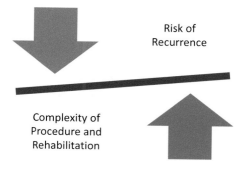

Risk of
Recurrence

Complexity of
Procedure and
Rehabilitation

Fig. 9.5 Patient-centric Dupuytren's care decision making

general or regional anaesthesia because of the complexities of the anaesthesia, surgery and post-operative programme. Nevertheless, this should be discussed during informed consent. Wide awake fasciectomy should form part of a logical, risk-stratified and evidence-based approach to Dupuytren's contracture (Fig. 9.6).

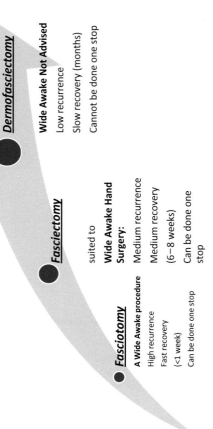

Fig. 9.6 Wide awake fasciectomy in context

OSWA Hand Surgery: Summary

Our experience with wide awake hand surgery in the United Kingdom over the last 15 years has concentrated on utilising the advantages of the wide awake approach to enable one-stop surgery and rehabilitation [5, 6]. The patient described here, like all our patients, was offered an OSWA patient-centric pathway. This involves an exchange of information pre-operatively, with the surgeon assessing the patient's suitability for OSWA and providing all the relevant information the patient requires to focus the clinical consultation and informed consent; patient information videos for informed consent and for rehabilitation instruction, via the Web, YouTube or via our bespoke patient apps; and online pre- and post-operative scoring to enable audit and governance.

Patient Centricity

Increasingly, the role of the patient-centric approach to healthcare is recognised as beneficial [11] and through OSWA and wide awake hand surgery we believe hand surgeons can deliver patient-centric care for Dupuytren's patients. In this context the modern Dupuytren's pathway as well as surgeon should

- Empower the patient by distilling relevant, focussed and impartial patient education materials (video).
- Provide such information in a range of multimedia formats and via the web, mobile applications and social media.
- Use the above to promote hand health for Dupuytren's patients.
- Utilise modern technology to provide the most efficient, streamlined patient pathway.
- Centre the patient in a surgical and rehabilitative experience, supported by online rehabilitation and monitoring.

Appendix on Wide Awake Anaesthesia: Key Points to Wide Awake Fasciectomy

Local Anaesthetics

- Local anaesthetics disrupt the inflow of sodium through channels in the membranes of neurones.
- They work better in smaller and rapidly firing nerves.
- This is why in wide awake hand surgery the pain fibres are invariably blocked whilst motor (movement) fibres are usually unaffected. Thus, our patients can benefit from pain-free surgery whilst feeling touch and being able to move the fingers and hand.
- This also means the wide awake hand surgeon can re-assess the hand during the procedure, with active movement.

Dosage Information as a Guide Only

Please see our principal source, http://www.ncbi.nlm.nih.gov/pmc/articles/PMC3403589.

- The maximum dose of lignocaine without adrenaline is 3 mg/kg.
- The maximum dose of lignocaine with adrenaline is 7 mg/kg.
- Thus, in a 70-kg patient, do not use more than

    – 20 ml of 1 % plain lignocaine or
    – 10 ml of 2 % plain lignocaine or
    – 48 ml of 1 % lignocaine with adrenaline or
    – 24 ml of 2 % lignocaine with adrenaline

Patients Not Suitable for Wide Awake Surgery

The only absolute contraindication is local anaesthetic allergy, which is rare. If there is any doubt that a patient may have a local anaesthetic allergy, he should be referred to an allergy specialist for evaluation and surgery should not be performed.

Rather than having a true allergy, patients are more likely to faint or to react to adrenaline (either their own adrenaline or that administered—adrenaline is a beta-1 adrenergic agonist). In our experience with wide awake hand surgery over 15 years, we have not encountered a patient who was confirmed to have a local anaesthetic allergy.

The least allergenic local anaesthesia would be an alternate amide such as prilocaine; use it without adrenaline and use a single-use vial (with no preservative).

If there are any doubts, postpone the surgery and refer to an allergy specialist.

Vasopressors

Vasopressors, such as low-dose adrenaline, for instance, at 1:200,000, are commonly used in wide awake hand surgery to provide constriction of blood vessels and hence minimise bleeding by activating alpha-1 adrenergic receptors. In addition to minimising bleeding in the operative field, low-dose adrenaline delays anaesthetic absorption, enabling pain-free surgery for more complex procedures. Delayed absorption of local anaesthetics reduces the risk for systemic toxicity and prolongs the duration of anaesthesia.

Low-Dose Adrenaline Contraindications Within Our Practice

Absolute

- Tricyclic and monoamine oxidase inhibitor antidepressants
- Digoxin
- Thyroid hormone
- Sympathomimetics used for weight control or attention deficit disorders
- Stimulant drug abuse (e.g., cocaine)
- Documented prior clinical problems with finger circulation or vascular supply to hand/upper limb
- Allergy (see above)

- Patient's expression at informed consent he or she wishes to avoid use of low-dose adrenaline in his or her case *for whatever reason*

Relative

- Cardiovascular disease
- Hypertension
- Vascular disease
- History of hand/upper limb circulatory problems (e.g., Raynaud's syndrome, vibration-induced white finger
- Beta blockers

Best Advice with Regards to Low-Dose Adrenaline Injection from Our Practice

- If you have any doubt, use plain local anaesthesia. Via anatomical dissection and intermittent firm point pressure with a rolled swab, any bleeding can be controlled without vasopressor use.
- The peak vasoconstrictor action/absorption of adrenaline is around 5 minutes after the injection and tails off each minute after this; hence, manage the risk of injury to the neurovascular structures or tendon mechanism accordingly. This is why we advocate straight incisions (see the section entitled 'Discussion') with Z-plasty as required (at the end of the procedure, deferred to a second stop or not done at all).

References

1. Lalonde D. How the wide awake approach is changing hand surgery and hand therapy: inaugural AAHS sponsored lecture at the ASHT meeting, San Diego, 2012. J Hand Ther. 2013;26(2):175–8. doi:10.1016/j.jht.2012.12.002. Epub 2013 Jan 5.
2. Nelson R, Higgins A, Conrad J, Bell M, Lalonde D. The wide-awake approach to Dupuytren's disease: fasciectomy under local anesthetic with epinephrine. Hand (N Y). 2010;5(2):117–24. doi:10.1007/s11552-009-9239-y. Epub 2009 Nov 10.

3. Bismil Q, Bismil M, Bismil A, Neathey J, Gadd J, Roberts S, Brewster J. The development of one-stop wide-awake Dupuytren's fasciectomy service: a retrospective review. JRSM Short Rep. 2012;3(7):48. doi:10.1258/shorts.2012.012050. Epub 2012 Jul 23.
4. Robbins TH. Dupuytren's contracture: the deferred Z-plasty. Ann R Coll Surg Engl. 1981;63(5):357–8.
5. Wakai A, Winter DC, Street JT, Redmond PH. Pneumatic tourniquets in extremity surgery. J Am Acad Orthop Surg. 2001;9(5):345–51.
6. Crews JC, Hilgenhurst G, Leavitt B, Denson DD, Bridenbaugh PO, Stuebing RC. Tourniquet pain: the response to the maintenance of tourniquet inflation on the upper extremity of volunteers. Reg Anesth. 1991;16(6):314–7.
7. Denkler K. Dupuytren's fasciectomies in 60 consecutive digits using lidocaine with epinephrine and no tourniquet. Plast Reconstr Surg. 2005;115(3):802–10.
8. Achar S, Kundu S. Principles of office anesthesia: part I. Infiltrative anesthesia. Am Fam Physician. 2002;66(1):91–5.
9. Bismil M, Bismil Q, Harding D, Harris P, Lamyman E, Sansby L. Transition to total one-stop wide-awake hand surgery service-audit: a retrospective review. JRSM Short Rep. 2012;3(4):23. doi:10.1258/shorts.2012.012019. Epub 2012 Apr 16.
10. Teo I, Lam W, Muthayya P, Steele K, Alexander S, Miller G. Patients' perspective of wide-awake hand surgery—100 consecutive cases. J Hand Surg Eur Vol. 2013;38(9):992–9. doi:10.1177/1753193412475241. Epub 2013 Jan 24.
11. Phaneuf M. The patient-centered approach, a humanistic pathway for care. Rev Infirm. 2014;201:36–8.

References for Appendix

Becker DE, Reed KL. Local anesthetics: review of pharmacological considerations. Anesth Prog. 2012;59(2):90–101. doi:10.2344/0003-3006-59.2.90. PMID: 22822998, quiz 102–3. Review.
Reed KL, Malamed SF, Fonner AM. Local anesthesia part 2: technical considerations. Anesth Prog. 2012;59(3):127–36. doi:10.2344/0003-3006-59.3.127. PMID: 23050753, quiz 137. Review.

Chapter 10
Surgical Open Palm (McCash) Technique

Panayotis N. Soucacos, Zinon Kokkalis, Aristides B. Zoubos, and Elizabeth O. Johnson

Case Presentation

A 44-year-old male presented to the Orthopedic Clinic with skin pitting and thickening, a rope like swelling in his palm, and an inability to fully straighten the ring and little fingers of his right hand. The patient noted that this had progressed over the last 18 months. The patient was a car mechanic with a history of several previous minor hand injuries attributed to his manual labor. The patient was a heavy smoker and had no other medical history of note. Physical examination showed flexion contractures of the

P.N. Soucacos, MD, FACS (✉) • A.B. Zoubos, MD
The "Panayotis N. Soucacos" Orthopaedic Research & Education Center,
Attikon University Hospital, National & Kapodistrian University of Athens,
Rimini 1, 124 62 Haidari, Athens, Greece
e-mail: psoukakos@ath.forthnet.gr

Z. Kokkalis, MD
Department of Orthopaedics, School of Medicine, University of Patras,
Patras, Greece

E.O. Johnson, PhD
Department of Anatomy, School of Medicine, National & Kapodistrian
University of Athens, 75 Mikras Asias Str. 11572 Goudi, Athens, Greece
e-mail: elizabethojohnson@gmail.com

© Springer International Publishing Switzerland 2016   137
M. Rizzo (ed.), *Dupuytren's Contracture*,
DOI 10.1007/978-3-319-23841-8_10

proximal interphalangeal joints, palpable nodules on the volar aspect of all proximal phalanges, and palpable cords to his lateral three digits. The flexion contracture was 42° and 62° at the meta-carpophalangeal (MCP) joint and proximal interphalangeal (PIP) joint, respectively, of the ring finger. The Orthopedic Surgeon diagnosed Dupuytren's disease and advised surgical treatment with an open palmar fasciectomy (McCash technique).

Diagnosis/Assessment

The patient demonstrated the typical presentation of Dupuytren's disease with nodules and pretendinous cords in the palm, which results in flexion contractures in the metacarpophalangeal and interphalangeal joints at the base of the ring and small fingers [1, 2]. Nodules are a pathognomonic sign of early disease and tend to be located just proximal or distal to the distal palmar crease and in the proximal segment of the digits, most frequently the ring and/or small finger. While nodules can present at the base of the thumb, they were absent in this particular patient. Pits and folds that form by the attachment of the diseased fascia to the skin are frequently mistaken for nodules. The cords observed in the patient suggest that the disease is still in early stages. The cords are palpable proximal and distal to the nodules as the contracture begins.

While a notable contracture is present in ring and little fingers, the fist of the disease hand appears normal. In addition the digits tend to lack extension (Fig. 10.1). In general, the digitus annularis of finger IV and finger V are affected the majority of times.

The disease, which occurs most commonly in middle-age males, is characterized by fibroblast proliferation and collagen deposition in the palmar aponeurosis and its digital prolongations resulting in a contraction. While the patient's history did not indicate a family history (compatible with an autosomal dominant pattern of inheritance), he was a heavy smoker. Smoking along with alcohol intake and diabetes mellitus has been associated with the disease [1–3]. The association with smoking is related to microvascular impairment which can be further augmented in combination

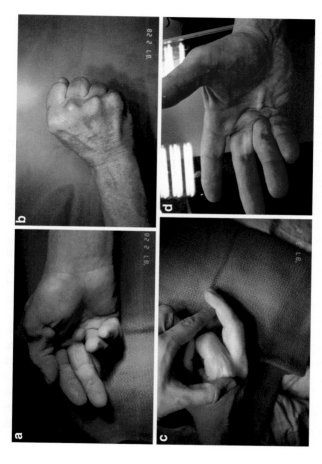

Fig. 10.1 Preoperative view showing flexion contracture of the ring and little finger (**a**). While the fist of the patient appears normal (**b**), the patient is unable to fully extend the digit (**c**). Palpable cords in lateral digits are a common feature (**d**)

with alcoholism. While trauma has not been considered a primary cause of Dupuytren, the fact that the patient has had several minor injuries to his hand related to heavy manual labor may be a contributing factor.

Management

While there are various nonoperative treatment options including Dimethyl sulfoxide massaging, ultrasonic therapy along with passive stretching exercises, splinting, steroids, enzymatic fasciotomy, collagenase enzymatic fasciotomy, among others, the surgeon opted for surgical management because the contracture of the MCP joint was greater than 30° which negatively affected the patients normal work routine. While there are no absolute indications for surgery, surgery is indicated for relief from bothersome contracture, >30° contracture at the MCP joint, any degree of contracture at the PIP joint, and the presence of painful nodules (relative indication).

There are several surgical options available to the surgeon. Local excision of the nodule, however, is rarely necessary, as nodules tend to recur. Fasciotomy to release the MCP flexion by division of the cord in the palm is often favored since the procedure is minimal with few complications, and allows for immediate MCP joint improvement with negligible postoperative disability. On the other hand, fasciotomy does not remove nodules, is less effective in correcting PIP contractures, and is associated with frequent recurrence of the disease. The most common surgical procedures are regional fasciectomy to excise all the diseased fascia and extensive fasciectomy, which excises all of the diseased fascia, as well as the potentially disease fascia. Various fasciectomy procedures have been devised, including percutaneous needle fasciotomy, open palm technique, Gonzales interpositional skin grafts, Hueston's dermofasciectomy, PIP joint release, among others [4–6]. While fasciectomy results in a decreased chance of recurrence, it entails excision of the aponeurosis and all the cords, regardless of their involvement, resulting in increased postoperative complications.

The patient was surgically managed with an open palmar fasciectomy (McCash technique) under axillary nerve block and high humeral tourniquet [7]. The rationale of using the method was to provide the surgeon with a direct view of the pathology and avoid complications, such as hematoma formation and skin necrosis from skin suture under tension, therefore ensuring adequate blood supply for the healing process [8–11]. Moreover, satisfactory results have been reported with this technique including less pain, better motion and low complication rate including hematoma, skin necrosis, and infection [8–13].

With the McCash open palm technique, fascia is excised through transverse incisions under axillary nerve block and high humeral tourniquet on an outpatient basis. The cords were approached using a z-shaped palmar incision followed by a crossing transverse incision (Fig. 10.2). Removal of the affected tissue through the transverse incision in the region of the distal palmar crease allows for the correction of the flexion deformity of the PCP joint. When necessary, another transverse incision can be made proximally to the first to further facilitate tissue resection. Once the neurovascular elements are meticulously dissected, then complete excision of the scar tissue and cords is performed. The palmar incision is left open and allowed to heal by secondary intention, which may take up to 6 weeks. Note: the palmar incisions are left open, but the phalangeal incisions are closed. While the transverse incisions are left open and allowed to granulate, occasionally they can be skin grafted with a full thickness skin graft (Fig. 10.3)

The wound is covered with Vaseline dressing and digits splinted in extension. Antibiotic prophylaxis with a second generation cephalosporin and NSAIDs are administered for 2–4 days, with a change of dressing after the first week and every 4–6 days thereafter. Physiotherapy is initiated 7 days postoperatively, and full activity is allowed 3 weeks postoperatively. Stitches are removed about 2 weeks postoperatively.

Outcome

The patient had excellent results. The wound healed with 8 weeks and sensory evaluation revealed no permanent numbness (Fig. 10.4). The average period for wound healing has been reported to be 40 days following the open hand technique [14].

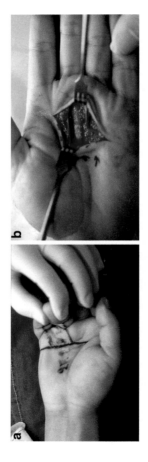

Fig. 10.2 The transverse palmar incision (**a**), and extension of incision to involved digits. Intraoperative view (**b**)

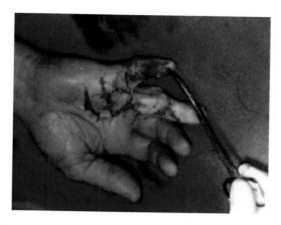

Fig. 10.3 Immediate postoperative view. Note the wound is left open

At a follow-up of 2 years, the MCP joint contracture improved to 1.8°, and the PIP joint contracture improved to 7.1°. This is similar to the finding of Lubahn [9, 15] who reported that 20 % of the patients experience residual contracture compared to 42 % observed in patients treated by suturing the operative wounds.

No complications were encountered in the present case. The absence of infection is attributed to the appropriate wound dressing and close patient monitoring. In general, patients treated with the open hand technique result in a less painful postoperative period, better mobility of the digits, and a lower rate of complications [10].

Literature Review

Satisfactory results have been reported with the McCash technique, with less pain, better motion, and a low complication rate, compared to other methods, which include hematomas, skin necrosis, and infection. The McCash open palm technique is favored for advanced disease states, especially diabetics, and is preferred for patients with multiple involvement.

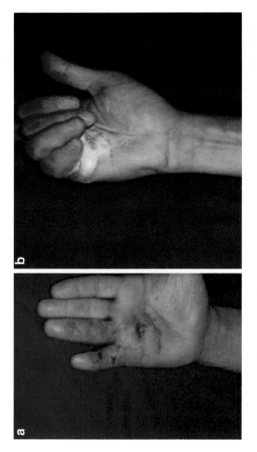

Fig. 10.4 Six weeks postoperative view, showing digit extension (**a**) and flexion (**b**)

The various options available to treat Dupuytren's disease have had variable results. In general, final outcome after surgery tends to be worse in patients who have an early onset of the disease or severe PIP joint involvement. To date, no medical strategy has demonstrated effective long-term results in halting or reversing the progression of the contracture [11, 12, 16].

Hence, despite the relatively favorable outcomes with the McCash technique, the surgeons must stress to their patients that surgery is not a cure for the disease, but a means of relieving some of the disability associated with the disease.

Clinical Pearls/Pitfalls

- Open wounds frequently lead to infection, especially in patients with abnormal healing. This stresses the importance of appropriate wound dressing and close monitoring.
- Adherence to strict rehabilitation program is essential.
- Postoperative extension splinting is mandatory.
- When contractures are corrected, a gap of 3–4 cm may be present.
- Common intraoperative pitfall, inadvertent division of a digital nerve (Loupe magnification and patience are essential).
- During dissection of neurovascular bundle, note that the nerve usually travels deeper into fascia in the area of the diseased fascia mass. (Do not excise any tissue until the digital nerve has been identified on both sides of the excision zone.)

References

1. Hu FZ, Nystrom A, Ahmed A, Palmquist M, Dopico R, Mossberg I, Gladitz J, Rayner M, Post JC, Ehrlich GD, Preston RA. Mapping of an autosomal dominant gene for Dupuytren's contracture to chromosome 16q in a Swedish family. Clin Genet. 2005;68:424–9.
2. Renard E, Jacques D, Chammas M, et al. Increased prevalence of soft tissue hand lesions in type 1 and type 2 diabetes mellitus: various entities and associated significance. Diabete Metab. 1994;20:513.

3. Burge P, Hoy G, Regan P, Milne R. Smoking, alcohol and the risk of Dupuytren's contracture. J Bone Joint Surg Br. 1997;79:296–310.

4. Roush TF, Stern PJ. Results following surgery for recurrent Dupuytren's disease. J Hand Surg Am. 2000;25(2):291–6.

5. Bainbridge C, Dahlin LB, Szczypu PP, Cappelleri JC, Guérin D, Gerber RA. Current trends in the surgical management of Dupuytren's disease in Europe: an analysis of patient charts. Eur Orthop Traumatol. 2012;3: 31–41.

6. Boyer MI, Gelberman RH. Complications of the operative treatment of Dupuytren's disease. Hand Clin. 1999;15:161–6.

7. McCash CR. The open palm technique in Dupuytren's contracture. Br J Plast Surg. 1964;17:271–80.

8. Zachariae L. Operation for Dupuytren's contracture by the method of McCash. Acta Orthop Scand. 1970;41:433–8.

9. Lubahn J. Open palm technique and soft tissue coverage in Dupuytren's Disease. Hand Clin. 1999;15:127–36.

10. Schneider L, Hankin F, Eisenberg T. A review of the open palm method. J Hand Surg Am. 1986;11:23–7.

11. Gelberman R, Panagis J, Hergenroder P, Zakaib GS. Wound complications in the surgical management of Dupuytren's contracture: a comparison of operative incisions. Hand. 1982;14:248–53.

12. Mavrogenis AF, Spyridonos SG, Ignatiadis IA, Antonopoulos D, Papagelopoulos PJ. Partial fasciectomy for Dupuytren's contractures. J Surg Orthop Adv. 2009;18(2):106–10.

13. Zoubos AB, Stavropoulos NA, Babis GC, Mavrogenis AF, Kokkalis ZT, Soucacos PN. The McCash technique for Dupuytren's disease: our experience. Hand Surg. 2014;19:61–7.

14. Skoff HD. The surgical treatment of Dupuytren's contracture: a synthesis of techniques. Plast Reconstr Surg. 2004;113(2):540–4.

15. Lubahn JD, Lister GD, Wolfe T. Fasciectomy and Dupuytren's disease: a comparison between the open-palm technique and wound closure. J Hand Surg Am. 1984;9A(1):53–8.

16. Gilpin D, Coleman S, Hall S, Houston A, Karrasch J, Jones N. Injectable collagenase Clostridium histolyticum: a new nonsurgical treatment for Dupuytren's disease. J Hand Surg Am. 2010;35:2027–38.

Suggested Readings

Cools H, Verstreken J. The open palm technique in the treatment of Dupuytren's Disease. Acta Orthop Belg. 1994;60:413–20.

Lubahn JD. Open-palm technique and soft-tissue coverage in Dupuytren's disease. Hand Clin. 1999;15:127–36.

Schneider LH, Hankin FM, Eisenberg T. Surgery of Dupuytren's disease: a review of the open palm method. J Hand Surg Am. 1986;11:23–7.

Chapter 11
Treatment of Dupuytren's Contracture with Dermofasciectomy

Nathan A. Monaco, C. Liam Dwyer, and John D. Lubahn

History

A 59-year-old retired right hand dominant male with history of Dupuytren's contracture was evaluated in our Hand Clinic for recurrent disease in the left palm (Fig. 11.1). Five years prior to evaluation, both hands had been treated with limited fasciectomy and primary wound closure at an outside facility. He was asymptomatic for 4 years when he began to complain of difficulty gripping a golf club. He reported disease in both hands, but was only symptomatic on the left. Interestingly, recurrent disease on the right small finger had led to a PIPJ flexion contracture which he believed helped him better grip a golf club and improved his game.

N.A. Monaco, MD (✉) • C.L. Dwyer, MD • J.D. Lubahn, MD
Department of Orthopaedic Surgery, UPMC-Hamot,
201 State Street, Erie, PA 16550, USA
e-mail: monacona@upmc.edu; jdlubahn@jdlubahn.com

© Springer International Publishing Switzerland 2016   147
M. Rizzo (ed.), *Dupuytren's Contracture*,
DOI 10.1007/978-3-319-23841-8_11

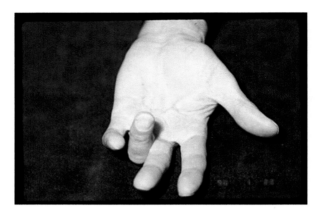

Fig. 11.1 A 59-year-old right hand dominant male with left ring and small finger involvement

Physical Exam Findings

On examination, the patient was a thin-statured, otherwise healthy appearing man in good health. He had a painful cord in the palm of the left hand overlying the ring finger metacarpal, with extension to the long and small fingers. There was a fixed MPJ contracture of the ring finger measuring 40°, with active flexion to 70°. Flexion contractures were measured at 10° and 20° at the long and small finger MPJs, respectively. A PIP contracture of the right ring finger was also noted and measured at 20°, with active flexion to 90°. Neurovascular examination demonstrated distal digital sensation intact to light touch with two-point discrimination measuring 5 mm in each digit. Grip strength was diminished on the left compared to the right dominant extremity, although he did demonstrate normal sensation in both hands on Semmes-Weinstein filament testing.

Treatment Options

Various options exist for treatment of recurrent Dupuytren's disease ranging from nonoperative care with collagenase injection to needle aponeurotomy or segmental aponeurectomy as described by Moermans [1, 2]. More invasive procedures such as fasciectomy and wound closure, or leaving the wound open as described by McCash [3], are also options. Dermofasciectomy, another type of invasive procedure, involves surgical excision of diseased skin and palmar fascia down to the level of the flexor tendon sheath. The defect in the palm is then covered by a full thickness skin graft harvested from a non-hair bearing area of the skin.

Some authors advocate collagenase clostridium histolyticum (CCH) injection to treat recurrent Dupuytren's disease, as it can potentially help lessen both the small joint contractures and the previous surgical scar [4]. However, no long-term outcome data is currently available for treatment of recurrent Dupuytren's contracture with CCH. Furthermore, tendon rupture is a risk following injection with collagenase if appropriate consideration is not given to needle placement [5]. Injection of CCH even in primary contracture cases has been found to demonstrate joint recurrence rates of up to 35 % at 3-year follow-up [6]. Cost can be an important consideration for many patients. A significant financial burden can be placed on the patient with Dupuytren's seeking treatment with CCH. In one cost-analysis study, a single injection of CCH was estimated at $1000 [7].

Percutaneous needle fasciotomy (PNF), also known as needle aponeurotomy, has also been offered as a therapeutic treatment option for recurrent Dupuytren's. Proponents of this technique argue that it is minimally invasive, it can potentially hasten recovery time compared to open techniques, and it is associated with an overall low complication rate [8]. In addition, the procedure may potentially be advantageous in that it can be performed in the office or under local anesthesia. Despite several advantages of PNF, patients can still have difficulty with recurrence. A study by van Rijssen utilized PNF to manage 40 digital cases of recurrent Dupuytren's and demonstrated a recurrence rate of up to 50 % at 4-year follow-up [9].

Segmental aponeurectomy (SA) aims at correcting contracture deformity by creating multiple areas of discontinuity in the palmar aponeurosis through small (1–2 cm) semilunar skin incisions. While many authors have contributed to the conceptual formation of the technique, Moermans described it in 1991 [1]. Initially the technique was developed as a less invasive means of correcting deformity while limiting the postoperative discomfort found after widespread dissection. Other surgeons have subsequently used segmental releases of the palmar fascia through transverse incisions to treat Dupuytren's [10]. Follow-up studies for many of these approaches, however, have demonstrated recurrence rates up to 38 %, while also reporting instances of iatrogenic nerve injury [2].

Partial or limited fasciectomy (LF) has been used for both primary and recurrent disease. Limited is a relative term, though, as this technique is one of the more invasive approaches to Dupuytren's contracture management. The procedure is "limited" in the sense that only macroscopic disease tissue is surgically excised. This stands in contrast to the historical approach of totally or completely removing the entire palmar fascia [11]. Total, or radical fasciectomy, is now often avoided due to morbidity concerns [12]. While LF has shown to reliably improve deformity, this approach is not without complication [13]. Nerve injury, hematoma, infection, worsening of the preoperative deformity, and circulatory compromise have all been reported [14].

Treatment Chosen

The patient being presented was treated in 1990, prior to the release of collagenase and prior to needle aponeurotomy or segmental aponeurectomy being widely accepted. Dermofasciectomy at the time was widely accepted as the state-of-the-art treatment for recurrent Dupuytren's disease. While dermofasciectomy carries with it the risk of donor site morbidity and longer healing time for the skin graft to take, full thickness skin grafting offers the potential advantage of lowering the risk for disease recurrence [15]. It was primarily to minimize the risk of recurrence that the decision was made to proceed with dermofasciectomy.

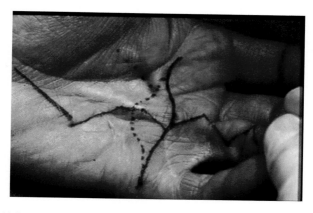

Fig. 11.2 Proposed preoperative markings for a planned incision and treatment of skin excision with skin grafting. The previous fasciectomy surgical sites can also be visualized

With the patient in the supine position, satisfactory general anesthesia was induced. A sterile tourniquet was applied to the upper extremity and inflated to 250 mmHg after routine prepping and draping of the arm. The surgical approach involved placing a Brunner-style, zig-zag incision over the palm (Fig. 11.2). Excision of the superficial skin took place in ellipse fashion centered over the distal palmar crease of the previously marked site (Fig. 11.3). Careful dissection was carried out with a combination of 15-blade scalpel and tenotomy scissors in a proximal to distal fashion. The final objective was removal of all deep palmar fascia with preservation of the neurovascular bundle. Once adequate resection of diseased tissue was achieved, the long ring and small fingers could be brought into full extension at the MPJ. The ring finger was then secured with a lead hand to maintain the PIP and MCP joint in maximal extension for graft application. A minimal residual PIPJ contracture was felt to be acceptable. Next, a full thickness skin graft was harvested from the medial brachium (Fig. 11.4a). The graft was de-fatted and sutured into place of the defect with 5-0 nylon suture. Tie-over sutures were also used to secure the graft. Donor site closure was performed using 5-0 nylon suture thrown in a simple-interrupted manner (Fig. 11.4b). The tourniquet was deflated prior to final closure and meticulous hemostasis was

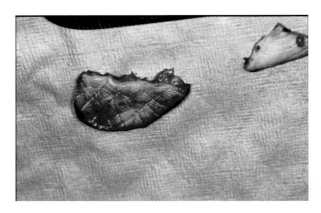

Fig. 11.3 Full thickness skin was excised from the diseased left palmar surface

obtained with bipolar electrocautery to limit potential hematoma complications. A soft tissue dressing was then applied along with a static splint maintaining the hand in the safe position. Once the graft was completely healed, the sutures were removed and the patient was started in a formal hand therapy program which included nighttime splinting and gentle active motion.

Clinical Course

This patient's postoperative course was free of any complications. At the 3-month follow-up visit, there were no signs of recurrence or disease extension. The patient demonstrated full extension and flexion of the MPJs of the long ring and small fingers after healing of the skin graft (Fig. 11.5a, b). A 10° PIPJ contracture persisted in the ring finger. The patient was satisfied with the results of his dermofasciectomy, specifically in that he was able to return to being an avid golfer.

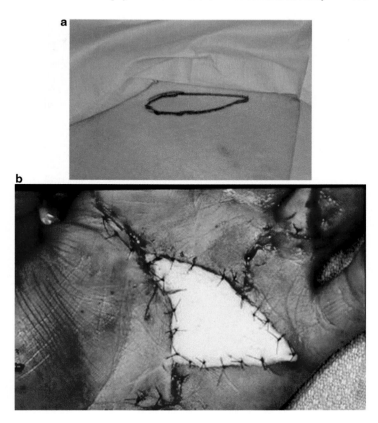

Fig. 11.4 (**a**) Donor site for full thickness skin graft. This was in an area void of hair, in the medial brachium. Alternative graft sites include skin inferior to the iliac crest and inner arm skin, with the key determinant being skin with similar characteristics between the donor and graft site. (**b**) Immediate postoperative appearance of left palm after application of full thickness skin graft

Discussion: Literature Review

The definition of "recurrence" of Dupuytren's disease varies among authors and short-term follow-up may limit our ability to accurately compare different treatment options. A systematic review concluded that at present, the evidence does not support

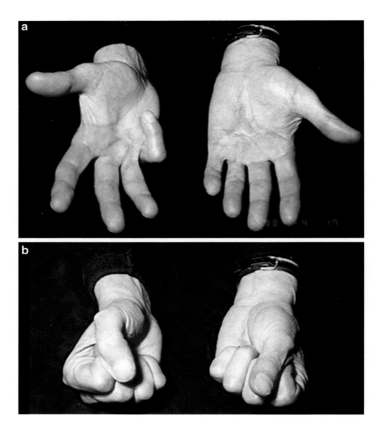

Fig. 11.5 (**a**) Three months postoperative. Patient noted to have healing of skin graft with improvement and almost full extension. (**b**) Range of motion with full flexion, allowing the patient to return to golf

clear superiority of one treatment over another in terms of degree of initial correction and prevention of recurrent disease [16]. Early observations reported by Gordon [17] and Hueston [18] that recurrence does not occur under an area of skin grafting led many surgeons to recommend and perform dermofasciectomy. Ketchum and Hickson noted no recurrence in 36 hands at an average of 4-year follow-up after dermofasciectomy [19]. Noting similar results, other authors reported that dermofasciectomy with full thickness skin graft resulted in lower rates of recurrence of Dupuytren's contracture [20].

Indications for use of dermofasciectomy often include recurrent disease as well as aggressive forms associated with diffuse skin involvement as well as with so-called "Dupuytren's diathesis." Armstrong and colleagues agreed with Hueston's indications, utilizing dermofasciectomy in cases of Dupuytren's with widespread skin association [21]. Abe collaborated to develop a scoring system for evaluation of disease recurrence and extension [22]. Components of this scale include bilateral disease (1), previous small finger surgery (1), early onset (1), ectopic plantar (2) or knuckle fibrosis (2) and radial sided disease (2). Out of a possible nine total risk points, patients scoring four or higher according to this classification demonstrate an indication for dermofasciectomy [23]. Anwar, while championing a local skin flap for mild disease, conceded an indication for dermofasciectomy to manage either severe involvement or recurrent disease [24]. Heuston noted that surgically devitalized skin and longitudinal skin deformity in the palm following flexion deformity correction can also be considered indications for skin grafting [25].

Results of recurrence following dermofasciectomy, while promising, have not always matched Hueston's early findings. Armstrong et al. reported a recurrence rate of 11.6 % in 103 patients managed with dermofasciectomy over a mean 5.8-year follow-up period [21]. The authors suggested considering dermofasciectomy as a "subtotal preaxial amputation of the digit," with an emphasis on removing all tissue that may be responsible for contracture. This differs from Hueston's belief that it is merely the insertion of a full thickness skin graft that is the key component to Dupuytren's disease control. Brotherston, however, found no evidence of disease recurrence after dermofasciectomy at an average follow-up of 100 months in 34 patients [26]. Hall reported six cases of recurrence in a series of 90 digits (7 %) with 48-month follow-up [27], and Roy found seven recurrences in 100 cases (7 %) followed for 52 months post dermofasciectomy [28].

Only a few studies have attempted the difficult task of comparing dermofasciectomy to other operative techniques to manage recurrent Dupuytren's. Tonkin and colleagues compared 100 patients managed with either dermofasciectomy or fasciectomy [29].

At an average follow-up of 38 months, there were only three cases of recurrence in the skin graft group, compared to an overall rate of recurrence of 47% in the study. The authors argued that skin grafting , specifically interposition of dermal tissue following Dupuytren's excision, may limit recurrence in comparison to fasciectomy for recurrent Dupuytren's disease. Rouch and Stern compared results of 28 digits at median of 4-year follow-up in three treatment groups for recurrent Dupuytren's: limited fasciectomy, dermofasciectomy, and fasciectomy with local skin flaps [30]. These authors found that skin grafting did not limit postoperative contracture and the only statistically limited recurrence rate was found in the treatment group managed with a locally based flap. A definitive conclusion regarding superiority of the technique of fasciectomy with local flap coverage versus dermofasciectomy was unable to be reached due to heterogeneity among the study's treatment groups. One prospective trial randomized 90 digits in patients treated with fasciectomy plus skin grafting or fasciectomy plus local skin z-plasty [31]. At the 3-year follow-up, no difference was found in the recurrence rate of the skin grafts (13.6%) and Z-plasty (10.9%) group. In general, the available evidence currently suggests that there may still be a role for dermofasciectomy in the treatment of Dupuytren's disease, with particular utility in cases of recurrent disease.

Complication after use of dermofasciectomy may be significant. Reported complications following this technique range from mild skin irritation or transient digital neuropraxia to major skin necrosis and loss of the graft. Hematoma, skin necrosis, iatrogenic digital nerve, and vascular injury as well as infection have all been reported following dermofasciectomy [12]. Surgeons may be hesitant to use this technique, considering the risk of the skin graft not taking over a flexor tendon and/or the neurovascular bundle. Armstrong notes, however, that graft incorporation is usually successful unless both digital arteries have been damaged [21]. In addition to operative complications, there are also a number of associated surgical morbidities which may prove undesirable to the patient. Skoog noted patients undergoing radical fasciectomy complained of palm sensitivity, particularly when grasping heavy objects [11]. Because palmar sensitivity was a common complaint and a problem for Skoog's factory worker patient population, he recommended a more limited excision over total fasciectomy. Unfortunately, the risk for palmar sensitivity under the graft site remains with dermofasciectomy.

Minor subtleties between donor and recipient skin can lead to variations in the appearance of the graft, such as difference in color and/or the potential for hair growth. For this reason, it is important to harvest donor skin that has characteristics as similar as possible to the recipient site. Common donor sites include the proximal forearm (brachium), the inner upper arm, and redundant skin surrounding the iliac crest. The patient must be willing to accept a residual postoperative surgical scar at whatever donor site is ultimately chosen. In addition, the patient may have a longer recovery time following a grafting procedure when compared to alternative less invasive techniques.

Despite the potential for operative morbidity and complication, dermofasciectomy may offer the advantage of prevention of recurrent disease. If the technique is efficacious in preventing recurrence, the patient also benefits from avoiding additional surgery. This would be especially useful in an instance where the patient may be predisposed to recurrence.

The patient presented offers one possible scenario where dermofasciectomy may be a useful treatment option. This particular individual had already had one previous fasciectomy procedure. His disease and his contracture recurred, however, along with a functional deficit impairing his ability to participate in avocational activities. In such instances, fasciectomy and subsequent full thickness skin grafting is a technique that has been safely used and may help limit future disease recurrence. In the absence of available evidence supporting one superior technique, dermofasciectomy remains a viable surgical option in cases of recurrent Dupuytren's contracture.

Summary

Dermofasciectomy involves excision of skin that is intimately associated with underlying diseased palmar fascia in Dupuytren's contracture. In the void remaining after volar palm tissue excision, a full thickness skin graft is placed to limit disease recurrence. The dermofasciectomy technique may be especially useful in the setting of recurrent Dupuytren's disease or in cases with widespread contracture. Our patient demonstrates that in an appropriately selected individual, dermofasciectomy can be safely utilized to improve range of motion, strength, and overall hand function of an affected extremity.

References

1. Moermans JP. Segmental aponeurectomy in Dupuytren's disease. J Hand Surg Br. 1991;16B:243–54.
2. Moermans JP. Long-term results after segmental aponeurectomy for Dupuytren's disease. J Hand Surg Br. 1996;21:797–800.
3. McCash CR. The open palm technique in Dupuytren's contracture. J Plast Surg Br. 1964;17:271–80.
4. Denkler KA. Collagenase for recurrent dupuytren contracture with skin grafts. J Hand Surg Am. 2013;38(6):1264.
5. Zhang AY, Curtin CM, Hentz VR. Flexor tendon rupture after collagenase injection for Dupuytren contracture: case report. J Hand Surg Am. 2011;36(8):1323–5.
6. Peimer CA, et al. Dupuytren contracture recurrence following treatment with collagenase Clostridium histolyticum (CORDLESS Study): 3-year data. J Hand Surg Am. 2013;38(1):12–22.
7. Chen NC, Shauver MJ, Chung KC. Cost-effectiveness of open partial fasciectomy, needle aponeurotomy, and collagenase injection for Dupuytren's contracture. J Hand Surg Am. 2011;36A:1826–34.
8. Eaton C. Percutaneous fasciotomy for Dupuytren's contracture. J Hand Surg Am. 2011;36A:910–5.
9. van Rijssen AL, Werker PMN. Percutaneous needle fasciotomy for recurrent Dupuytren disease. J Hand Surg Am. 2012;37A:1820–3.
10. Shin EK, Jones NF. Minimally invasive technique for release of Dupuytren's contracture: segmental fasciectomy through multiple transverse incisions. Hand. 2011;6:256–9.
11. Skoog T. Dupuytren's contracture: pathogenesis and surgical treatment. Surg Clin North Am. 1967;47(2):433–44.
12. Henry M. Dupuytren's disease: current state of the art. Hand. 2014;9:1–8.
13. Denkler K. Surgical complications associated with fasciectomy for Dupuytren's disease: a 20-year review of the English literature. J Plast Surg. 2010;10:116–33.
14. Dias JJ, Braybrooke J. Dupuytren's contracture: an audit of the outcomes of surgery. J Hand Surg (Br). 2006;31(5):514–21.

15. Rizzo M, Stern PJ, Benhaim P, Hurst LC. Contemporary management of Dupuytren contracture. Instr Course Lect. 2014;63:131–42.
16. Becker GW, Davis TR. The outcome of surgical treatments for primary Dupuytren's disease—a systematic review. J Hand Surg Eur. 2010;35(8):623–6.
17. Gordon S. Dupuytren's contracture: recurrence and extension following surgical treatment. Br J Plast Surg. 1957;9:286–8.
18. Hueston JT. Digital Wolfe grafts in recurrent Dupuytren's contracture. Plast Reconstr Surg. 1962;29:342–4.
19. Ketchum LD, Hixson FP. Dermofasciectomy and full-thickness grafts in the treatment of Dupuytren's contracture. J Hand Surg. 1987;12A:659–63.
20. Varian JPW. Full thickness skin grafts in the management of recurrent Dupuytren's disease. In: Hueston JT, Tubiana R, editors. Dupuytren's disease. 2nd ed. London: Churchill Livingstone; 1985. p. 154–7.
21. Armstrong JR, Jurren JS, Logan AM. Dermofasciectomy in the management of Dupuytren's disease. J Bone Joint Surg [Br]. 2000;82-B:90–4.
22. Abe Y, Rokkaku T, Ofuchi S, et al. An objective method to evaluate the risk of recurrence and extension of Dupuytren's disease. J Hand Surg Br. 2004;29B:427–30.
23. Tubiana R. Surgical indications. In: Tubiana R, Leclercq C, Hurst LC, Badalamente MA, Mackin EJ, editors. Dupuytren's disease. London: Martin Dunitz; 2000. p. 218–22.
24. Anwar MU, Al Ghazal SK, Boome RS. The lateral digital flap for Dupuytren's fasciectomy at the proximal interphalangeal joint—a study of 84 consecutive patients. J Hand Surg (Eur). 2009;34E(1):90–3.
25. Hueston JT. Skin replacement in Dupuytren's contracture. In: Hueston JT, Tubiana R, editors. Dupuytren's disease. Edinburgh: Churchill Livingstone; 1974. p. 119–22.
26. Brotherston TM, Balakrishnan C, Milner RH, Brown HG. Long term follow-up of dermofasciectomy for Dupuytren's contracture. Br J Plast Surg. 1994;47:440–3.
27. Hall PN, Fitzgerald A, Sterne GD, Logan AM. Skin replacement in Dupuytren's disease. J Hand Surg. 1997;22-B:193–7.
28. Roy N, Sharma D, Mirza A, Fahmy N. Fasciectomy and full thickness skin grafting in Dupuytren's contracture. The fish technique. Acta Orthop Belg. 2006;72:678–82.
29. Tonkin MA, Burke FD, Varian JPW. Dupuytren's contractures: a comparative study of fasciectomy and dermofasciectomy in one hundred patients. J Hand Surg Br. 1984;9B:156–62.
30. Roush RF, Stern PJ. Results following surgery for recurrent Dupuytren's disease. J Hand Surg. 2000;25A:291–6.
31. Ullah AS, Dias JJ, Bhowal B. Does a 'firebreak' full-thickness skin graft prevent recurrence after surgery for Dupuytren's contracture? J Bone Joint Surg Br. 2009;91-B:374–8.

Chapter 12
Surgical Fasciectomy for Recurrent Disease

Ombretta Spingardi and Mario Igor Rosello

Case Presentation

A 72-year-old retired male presented 7 years after a fasciectomy
for Dupuytren's disease involving the fourth and the fifth finger
of his left hand. Four years after surgery, a new nodule appeared
into his left palm while a progressive retraction and joint stiffness
in the site of the previous surgery were already appreciable at
least 1 year after treatment (Fig. 12.1). He complained gradual
impairment of his left hand function and the stiffness of his left
finger.

O. Spingardi, MD (✉) • M.I. Rosello, MD
Department of Hand Surgery, San Paolo Hospital, via Genova 30,
Savona 17100, Italy
e-mail: ombretta.s@libero.it; info@chirurgiamanorossello.it

© Springer International Publishing Switzerland 2016
M. Rizzo (ed.), *Dupuytren's Contracture*,
DOI 10.1007/978-3-319-23841-8_12

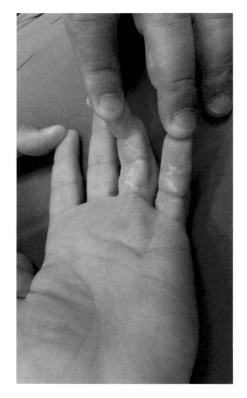

Fig. 12.1 Preoperative view of Dupuytren's recurrence with disease extension to palm; a retracting skin scar on the volar surface of DIP joint of fourth finger and PIP joint contracture of the fifth finger are appreciable

Physical Examination

Examination findings demonstrated a cord which coerced the PIP joint of the ring finger at 40° of flexion. Furthermore, the progressive skin retraction on the volar side of the DIP joint of the ring finger limited the motion of the finger and it was very bothering for the patient. In addition, he had a significant contracture of the small finger PIP joint with similar deficit of extension. His prior scars were nicely healed and he was neurovascularly intact. Given the severity of contracture, its progression, and the disability of the patient, intervention was warranted.

Treatment Options

Both operative and nonoperative treatment options can be considered for this condition. Office-based procedures include needle aponeurotomy and collagenase. In addition, operative interventions are an option. After lengthy deliberation of treatment options, surgical treatment with fasciectomy was decided upon as it afforded the opportunity to address both the diseased fascia as well as prior scar and capsular contracture.

The aims in this secondary surgery were to treat the digital Dupuytren's recurrence and its palmar extension and to correct the PIP joint stiffness and the skin scar retraction. These represent the main and more common problems coexisting in further treatment.

Management

As showed in Figs. 12.2 and 12.3, we used multiple "Z-plasties" to correct the scar retraction and to gain the volar opening after a meticulous dissection of neurovascular bundles at the fourth and fifth fingers and careful new aponeurotic tissue removal; at the same time a volar PIP joint arthrolysis by check-reins section has been done. All these procedures allowed to achieve the complete

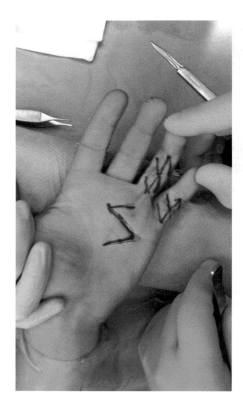

Fig. 12.2 Preoperative aspect. The Z-plasties are drawn to increase the skin length for a better wound coverage

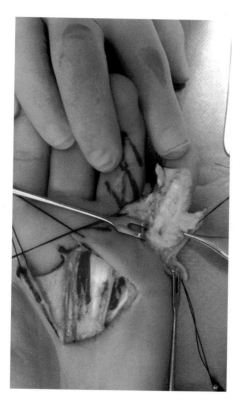

Fig. 12.3 Perioperative view. A careful research and dissection of neurovascular bundles is mandatory before treating the articular contracture

extension of the blocked joints. The patient started the active and passive motion immediately and 10 days after surgical treatment a corrective splint was put in place on the small finger to maintain the PIP extension.

Discussion

Defining the recurrence in Dupuytren's disease is very difficult because there is no consensus in world literature. Since the first disease descriptions and observations, many eminent authors made a lot of efforts to find an effective definition of this common consequence of its treatment.

Tubiana was among the first authors who tried to define the recurrence [1]. He defined recurrence as "the reappearance of Dupuytren contracture tissue in a zone previously operated." Hueston felt that reapparition of the smallest nodule constituted recurrence [2]. Gordon felt that recurrent disease in the same area defined recurrence [3]. Later, these definitions reappeared in the literature alternating with new other definitions by Gelberman [4] who felt that "the appearance of new fascial bands, determined by appearance and palpation, in an area where fasciectomy had been previously performed" was an appropriate definition of recurrence. Rombouts [5], Foucher [6], Adam [7], and many others [8] also described recurrence including some of the definitions previously reported.

The absence of consensus about recurrence definition is accompanied with confusion about rate of recurrence, which ranges from 2 to 86 % in the worldwide literature [4, 9, 10]. Kan et al. reported recurrence as either the return of nodules or cords in operated hand, the return of contraction with angular threshold between 1° and 50°, or patients self-reporting recurrence. It depends on many factors including intrinsic (the same disease, the patients' needs, the disease degree, and its extension) and extrinsic (surgical technique used). However, no surgical technique appears to be linked with more favorable recurrence rates. Open treatment (fasciectomy, aponeurectomy) has recurrence rates from 12 to 73 % [8], while Collagenase injection recurrence rates are 10 % for MCP joints contractures and 20° for PIP joints at 5 years [11]; the rates are higher after percutaneous needle fasciotomy: ranging from 58 % at 3 years and up to 100 % in other series [8, 12].

For these reasons in 2012, in Rome, an international consensus conference formed by 24 hand surgeons from 17 European countries tried to assess a definition of recurrence using the Delphi method [13, 14], which is a process of anonymous data collection from experts judgments. The conclusions of the consensus conference have been the following:

- The presence of a new nodule cannot be considered a recurrence.
- To assess an extension deficit, the measurement of the passive extension deficit of the treated joint must be used; the consensus has not been reached about the total passive extension deficit (TPED) measurement because it is not considered as precise as single joint measurement.
- The "time 0" definition, as the time when treatment results can be considered stable at follow-up, is the period between 6 weeks and 3 months after treatment.

Because of the confusion about recurrence in literature, it is mandatory a quantitative definition of recurrence: the occurrence of a new nodule can be considered a recurrence only after radical treatment (fasciectomy), not after fasciotomy, needle aponeurotomy, or CCH (Collagenase Clostridium histolyticum) injection. To evaluate the results after these treatments, it is better to measure the return of contracture in angular degrees: the presence of nodules or cords without finger contracture is not suggestive of recurrence. The consensus has also been reached about the Tubiana scale system ineffectiveness. It is preferable to measure the goniometric degrees of passive extension deficit of contracted joint: recurrence can be appreciated when the angle is greater than 20°.

As Tubiana described [15], it is mandatory to distinguish "true" recurrence from the so-called "pseudo-recurrence" such as situations of scar retraction after previous treatment, where bad skin scars arise after surgical incision or joint stiffness persisting after treatment. The differential diagnosis is easy whenever the retraction appears late, once good correction of previous deformities can be appreciated, when associated deformities were already present before surgery, and they have been only partially corrected by treatment. A discerning characteristic is that scar retraction lays in correspondence to skin scar, arises early (few weeks after treatment), and is usually stable over time. On the other hand, recurrence due to progression of Dupuytren's disease tends to occur later and doesn't necessarily run along the skin scar.

Literature Review

The papers with longest follow-up periods show that recurrence belongs to Dupuytren's natural evolution [16]: Tubiana said "The recurrence percentage increases in the time," observing a series of patients with a long follow-up (8–14 years) where only 34% of them didn't develop any recurrence; the others got different recurrence patterns, with (24%) or without (42%) functional impairment. The recurrence rate would increase in cases of multiple rays involvement (68% of patients of this series), in a longer follow-up period and in young patients: all the patients who were less than 45 years old before surgery developed the recurrence. This data supports the relationship between patients' young age and disease aggressiveness. Mantero [17] in 1983 published the longest follow-up casuistry (30 years) in Dupuytren's recurrence and observed that in 100% of patients who were suffering from epilepsy and chronic alcoholism, while the mean recurrence rate was 97% in patients affected by cardiac or respiratory disease, 52% in diabetic people, and 47% in patients with generic bad general conditions. Particularly, the recurrence rate was higher in the first 3–5 years follow-up (43%); 20–30 years after surgery, the mean rate was 77%. Mc Grouter [18] reached similar conclusions. The longer patients are followed, the higher the recurrence rate: almost all patients suffering from Dupuytren's disease will develop a recurrence if their survival time will allow them it.

Clinical Pearls/Pitfalls

We believe in fasciectomy as the best and most effective treatment for Dupuytren's recurrences, because this technique allows to treat also the associated deformities: joint contracture, skin scars. In accordance with literature we treat only the symptomatic cases with a significant deformity or impairment. The aim of the treatment is to treat all the anatomical elements involved.

To decrease any skin flap necrosis rate, the surgical approach consists always in broken incisions on the skin, as Bruner's incision; however, we prefer multiple "Z"-plasties because they will warrant a better coverage of surgical field during the suture, with "healthy" skin, and consequent scar lengthening: it makes gain more palm and digit opening, facilitating and improving the correction of joint retraction too. When the scar tissue is poor and the "Z"-plasties are not enough to cover the underlying tissues, the full-thickness skin graft harvested from the wrist or the medial face of the forearm is used (the so-called "firebreak" graft, even if it doesn't warrant any other recurrence reapparition [17]).

A subcutaneous careful dissection allows to identify and protect the neurovascular bundles, often dislocated from their original position or already damaged during the previous treatment: this is the most delicate phase of the surgical treatment. Their accidental section may be one of the most common operative complications.

As already discussed, in recurrence surgery the joint contracture is one of the problems to solve.

The possible causes of joint stiffness, beyond a new aponeurotic tissue presence (and which has to be removed), may be: longitudinal retraction of flexor tendon sheath, capsular and ligamentous PIP joint contracture, interosseous and extensor tendon apparatus decay (wreaking a boutonnière deformity). The treatment will be different for each one of these associated deformities: from a simple tenolysis with flexor sheath opening, until check-reins resection (in case of mild and recent joint contracture) or volar plate detachment associated with glenoid laminae of collateral ligaments section. The boutonnière deformity is secondary to volar dislocation of lateral extensor tendon bundles due to joint contracture followed by the elongation of the central bundle of extensor tendon;

the interosseous muscle is consequently locked at the lateral side of MCP joint.

After correction of these deformities, a temporary joint fixation is made by a K-wire that we put in place for about 3 weeks to maintain the satisfactory joint position.

Before skin closure a careful hemostasis is performed after tourniquet release and a suction drain is put in place. The pulpal refilling is monitored and, when few minutes after tourniquet removal the fingertip is not well vascularized, the K-wire is removed to avoid any excessive stretching of the vascular bundles. It will partially compromise the extension recovery of the joint but at least it will not threaten the finger survival.

Sometimes, whenever the tendon apparatus or neurovascular bundles cannot be covered by skin flaps of multiple "Z" plasties, their coverage is achieved by pedicled local flaps. In all the cases without deep tissues exposure the firebreak skin grafts are helpful; in one case where the most of the skin was useless after a wide debridement we used Integra®: in this case a longer and more intensive wound dressing program has been necessary, but no complication occurred.

The possible complications described in literature [19, 20] are commonly early, as problems in wound healing (hematoma, skin flaps partial necrosis), postoperative swelling, nerve injury, and infection. In addition, one can develop complex regional pain syndrome (CRPS), new recurrence, skin scar retraction, and joint stiffness (until "hook finger" deformity). Our experience in our hand surgery department agrees about these literature data. Particularly, we never observed any case of persisting digital ischemia requiring partial or total ray amputation.

A bulky dressing for 24 h is held in place and it will be replaced as soon as possible by a splint.

Although the literature is very limited in hand rehabilitation, a careful protocol program is very important after Dupuytren's treatment to maintain the surgical results [21–23] and in our clinical current practice we extend the same principles to Dupuytren's recurrence surgery. The main goals of rehabilitation are to promote the wound healing and to keep the joint release and to regain the joint motion at the same time. A too stressing exercise can compromise the corner flaps and the skin grafts, encourage the development of dystrophic or hypertrophic skin scar, and trigger vascular crisis (and subsequent sympathetic flare) because of a too aggressive stretch to neurovascular bundles. For these reasons, a too aggressive manual therapy associated with aggressive use of extension orthosis should be strongly avoided in the earliest reeducation program phase. Any tension on neurovascular bundles and skin repair must be abolished. A dorsal progressive dynamic splint with MCP joint at 35–45° of flexion and IP joints in relaxed extension is used whenever the preoperative PIP joint contracture was mild (<30°) and a simple release of check-reins allowed its satisfactory correction; but if the preoperative joint stiffness is hardly and strictly framed, and a more aggressive procedure on the joint is necessary to improve the contracture, we prefer a volar progressive static splint with silicone support, to treat the skin scar at the same time: a too drastic stretching of the volar surface of the finger would be too aggressive either for a satisfying quality of skin healing or the maintained recovery of extension of the joint. A careful program of skin scar massages is recommended and it starts as soon as possible, with parallel Coban's wraps use and silicone gel sheets local applications. This program is followed for at least 4–6 weeks.

References

1. Tubiana R, Leclerc C, Hurst LC, Badalamente MA, Mackin EJ, editors. Dupuytren's disease. 1st ed. London: Martin Dunitz Ltd.; 2000. p. 239–49.
2. Hueston JT. Recurrent Dupuytren's contracture. Plast Reconstr Surg. 1963;31:66–9.
3. Gordon S. Dupuytren's contracture: recurrence and extension following surgical treatment. Br J Plast Surg. 1957;9:286–8.
4. Gelberman RH, Amiel D, Rudolph RM, Vance RM. Dupuytren's contracture. An electron microscopic, biochemical and clinical correlative study. J Bone Joint Surg. 1980;62A:425–32.
5. Rombouts JJ, Noel H, Legrain Y, Munting E. Prediction of recurrence in the treatment of Dupuytren's disease: evaluation of histologic classification. J Hand Surg. 1989;14A:644–52.

6. Foucher G, Cornil C, Lenoble E. Open palm technique for Dupuytren's disease. A five-year follow-up. Ann Chir Main Memb Super. 1992;11:362–6.

7. Adam RF, Loynes RD. Prognosis in Dupuytren's disease. J Hand Surg. 1992;17A:312–7.

8. Werker PM, Pess GM, van Rijssen AL, Denkler K. Correction of contracture and recurrence rates of Dupuytren contracture following invasive treatment: the importance of clear definitions. J Hand Surg Am. 2012;37A:2095–105.

9. Becker GW, Davis TR. The outcome of surgical treatments for primary Dupuytren's disease—a systematic review. J Hand Surg Br. 2010;35:623–6.

10. Kan HJ, Verrijp FW, Huisstede BMA, Hovius ERS, van Nieuwenhoven CA, Selles RW. The consequences of different definitions for recurrence of Dupuytren's disease. J Plast Reconstr Aesthet Surg. 2013;66:95–103.

11. Hurst L. Dupuytren's contracture. In: Wolfe SW, Hotchkiss RN, Pederson WC, Kozin SH, editors. Green's operative hand surgery. 6th ed. Philadelphia: Elsevier Churchill-Livingstone; 2011. p. 141–58.

12. Foucher G, Medina J, Navarro R. Percutaneous needle aponeurotomy: complications and results. J Hand Surg (Br). 2003;28:427–31.

13. Dalkey N, Helmer O. An experimental application of the Delphi method to the use of experts. Manage Sci. 1963;9:458–67.

14. Felici N, Marcoccio I, Giunta R, Haerle M, Leclercq C, Pajardi G, Wilbrand S, Georgescu AV, Pess G. Dupuytren contracture recurrence project: reaching consensus on a definition of recurrence. Handchir Mikrochir Plast Chir. 2014;46:1–5.

15. Tubiana R. Traitement des récidives. In: Tubiana R, Hueston JT, editors. La maladie de Dupuytren, Monographies du Groupe d'études de la Main. 3rd ed. Paris: Expansion scientifique française; 1986. p. 149–53.

16. Tubiana R, Leclercq C. Les récidives dans la maladie de Dupuytren. In: Tubiana R, Hueston JT, editors. La maladie de Dupuytren, Monographies du Groupe d'études de la Main. 3rd ed. Paris: Expansion scientifique française; 1986. p. 203–7.

17. Mantero R, Ghigliazza GB, Bertolotti P, Bonanno F, Ferrari GL, Grandis C, Rossello I, Moretti F. Les formes récidivantes de la maladie de Dupuytren. In: Tubiana R, Hueston JT, editors. La maladie de Dupuytren, Monographies du Groupe d'études de la Main. 3rd ed. Paris: Expansion scientifique française; 1986. p. 208–9.

18. Mc Grouter D. Dupuytren's contracture. In: Green D, Hotchkiss RN, Pederson WC, et al., editors. Green's operative hand surgery. 5th ed. Edinburgh: Churchill-Livingstone; 1986. p. 159–85.

19. Michon J, Merle M. Difficultés et complications dans la chirurgie de la maladie de Dupuytren. In: Tubiana R, Hueston JT, editors. La maladie de Dupuytren, Monographies du Groupe d'études de la Main. 3rd ed. Paris: Expansion scientifique française; 1986. p. 181–90.

20. Henry M. Dupuytren's disease: current state of the art. Hand. 2014;9:1–8.

21. Evans RB. Therapeutic management of Dupuytren's contracture, Chapter 23. In: Skirve TM, Osterman AL, Fedorczyk JM, Amadio PC, editors. Rehabilitation of hand and upper extremity. 6th ed. Philadelphia: Elsevier Mosby; 2011. p. 281–8.
22. Jerosch-Herold C, Shepstone L, Chojnowski AJ, Larson D, Barrett E, Vaughan SP. Night-time splinting after fasciectomy or dermo-fasciectomy for Dupuytren's contracture: a pragmatic, multi-centre, randomized controlled trial. BMC Muscoloskelet Disord. 2011;12:136.
23. Jerosch-Herold C, Shepstone L, Chojnowski AJ, Larson D. Splinting after contracture release for Dupuytren's contracture (SCoRD): protocol for a pragmatic, multi-centre, randomized controlled trial. BMC Muscoloskelet Disord. 2008;9:62.

Chapter 13
Use of Dynamic External Fixator (Digit Widget) in Dupuytren's Contracture

Atanu Biswas and Anthony Smith

Introduction

Management of proximal interphalangeal (PIP) joint flexion contracture is one of the most challenging problems resulting from Dupuytren's disease. Progressive Dupuytren's disease causes a shortening of the palmar soft tissues thereby restricting extension of the PIP joint. This restriction of active extension at the PIP joint is due to shortening of pretendinous cord(s), checkrein ligament development, contracture of the collateral ligaments, scar contracture, or a combination of these abnormalities [1, 2]. Therapeutic interventions are aimed to relieve this restriction of motion caused by the flexion contracture as well as to maintain gains in active digit extension [3]. Nonoperative techniques such as serial splinting, casting, and stretching exercises have been used to offer gradual lengthening and softening of the contracted tissue [4–9]. These techniques exploit the increase in newly synthesized collagen

A. Biswas, MD, MS • A. Smith, MD (✉)
Mayo Clinic Hospital, 5779 East Mayo Boulevard, Phoenix, AZ 85054, USA
e-mail: biswas.atanu@mayo.edu; smith.anthony@mayo.edu

© Springer International Publishing Switzerland 2016
M. Rizzo (ed.), *Dupuytren's Contracture*,
DOI 10.1007/978-3-319-23841-8_13

due to increases in levels of the degradative enzymes, metalloproteinases, collagenase, and cathepsins B and L observed when gradual lengthening of the contracted soft tissue occurs [9]. Serial splinting and casting have limitations consisting of dorsal digital skin ischemia, pain, and potential ulceration if used on severe contractures [3]. The Digit Widget (Hand Biomechanics Lab, Inc., Sacramento, CA) was developed for treatment of severe PIP joint contractures while avoiding the soft tissue complications associated with serial casting and splinting.

The Digit Widget is a dynamic external fixator designed to provide an extension torque across the PIP joint for lengthening the palmar soft tissues in cases of severe Dupuytren's disease. The torque exerted by the Digit Widget is transmitted through the digital skeleton, thereby obviating any forces on the skin. The patient is able to retain full flexion of the digit while the Digit Widget is in place by releasing the traction produced by the device and actively flexing the digit. The patient can also adjust the amount of extension torque to provide the least amount of force needed for gradual joint extension while avoiding PIP joint inflammation and swelling from too much applied torque.

The indication for use of the Digit Widget is to restore the flexion-extension torque imbalance in any PIP joint flexion contractures. Dupuytren's disease is the most common diagnosis for placement of the Digit Widget; however, other diagnoses causing flexion contracture of the PIP joint can be considered for use of the Digit Widget to restore PIP extension. Patients with evidence of joint destruction such as in arthritis or trauma are not candidates for placement of the Digit Widget. Patients with unstable or subluxed PIP joints such as those with collateral ligament injuries are also not suitable for placement of the Digit Widget. One must also inquire about previous pulley injuries or release of checkrein ligaments as evidence of these will increase the flexion force along the moment arms of the PIP joint which could lead to recurrence with a worse contracture.

Those patients who are appropriate candidates for placement of the Digit Widget will keep the device on for approximately 6 weeks. During this time, the Digit Widget functions to gradually lengthen the palmar soft tissues and neurovascular bundle of the affected finger while simultaneously decreasing the flexion deformity of the PIP joint. The goal of treatment is to provide the least amount of torque to allow gradual decrease of the flexion deformity towards full correction by 6 weeks with a target improvement of up to 15° per week. Once the PIP joint is near full extension and the volar PIP joint is supple, the Digit Widget is removed. If the improvement with Digit Widget therapy plateaus before approaching full extension or if the palmar soft tissues of the PIP joint have evidence of residual symptomatic Dupuytren's nodules or noncompliant hypertrophic scarring, the Digit Widget is removed and operative fasciectomy is performed [2].

While the Digit Widget has been described as a 1-stage procedure involving excision of the Dupuytren's bands and nodules followed by placement of the device, a 2-stage approach has produced better results with regard to restoring active PIP joint extension [2, 5, 7, 10, 11]. Accurate Digit Widget application is performed with fluoroscopic guidance. The dorsal mid-longitudinal axis of the affected digit is marked (Fig. 13.1).

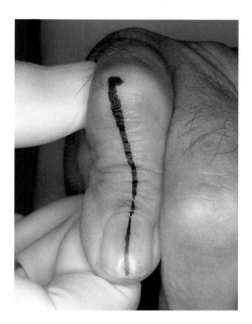

Fig. 13.1 Marking of the dorsal mid-longitudinal axis of the digit

Next, the PIP joint is radiographically identified using fluoroscopic guidance (Fig. 13.2a, b).

Once the PIP joint has been identified and marked, the locating drill guide placed on the mid-dorsum line just distal to the PIP joint (Fig. 13.3).

The locating drill guide is used to place a proximal and distal predrill pin under fluoroscopic guidance (Fig. 13.4a, b).

The distal predrill pin is then removed and replaced with a permanent distal screw followed by removal of the proximal predrill pin and subsequent replacement with a permanent proximal screw (Fig. 13.5a). Proper screw depth is confirmed with fluoroscopy (Fig. 13.5b).

After confirmation of permanent screw depth, the screw shrouds are cut and the drill guide is removed. The pin block is placed over the screws approximately 5 mm above the dorsal skin (Fig. 13.6).

The pin block is tightened in place with a hex wrench that is included in the Digit Widget kit. Also included in the Digit Widget kit is the connector assembly and rubber bands to set the torque force (Fig. 13.7). The connector assembly is attached to the Cuff. If the patient has hyperextension of the metacarpophalangeal (MP) joint while the Digit Widget is in place, an MP Flexion Strap is available to provide extension blocking of the MP joint.

As previously mentioned, the goal is to obtain full correction of the PIP joint flexion deformity by 6 weeks after placement of the Digit Widget. The patients are followed at weekly intervals and are monitored by plotting a graph of the change in range of motion as a function of time. The rubber bands, gauged as light, medium, and heavy, are changed daily and additional rubber bands are added if needed. Once five rubber bands of the same gauge are used simultaneously, a switch to a larger rubber band is made.

Frequent patient follow-up is required not only to monitor the results of distraction but also to monitor for potential complications. Since the Digit Widget is held in place to the middle phalanx by bone pins, the pins may serve as a tract for developing superficial or deep pin site infection. Thus, the patient should be educated on proper hygiene care of the device during the postoperative course. During distraction therapy, the patient should also be educated on adjusting the ideal torque force with the rubber bands.

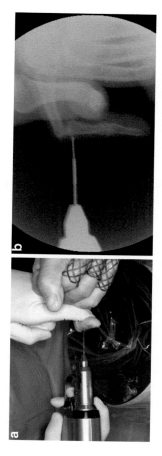

Fig. 13.2 (a) Identification of PIP joint with (b) fluoroscopic guidance

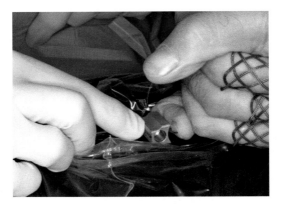

Fig. 13.3 Locating drill guide placement

If one applies too much torque on the PIP joint, the patient may experience pain, increased edema accompanied with swelling, inflammation, and possible decreased or loss of flexion in the PIP joint. Edema causing stiffness across the PIP joint will further undermine the effectiveness of the Digit Widget. Careful monitoring of the MP joint should also be addressed. The extension torque on the MP joint caused by PIP joint flexion contractures leads to MP joint hyperextension which reduces the efficiency of the Digit Widget [3]. This torque imbalance heavily trends toward MP joint hyperextension due to a reduced resting tension in the proximally translocated flexor digitorum superficialis and profundus tendons as well as an increased moment arm due to the dorsal dislocation of the extensor tendon off the metacarpal head. The result is a limitation of proximal excursion of the extensor tendon and its central slip. The net effect is inefficient mechanics required for PIP joint extension. Therefore, critical to achieving long-term active PIP joint extension after reversal of the PIP contracture is to restore central slip tension and excursion. If one identifies excessive hyperextension in the MP joint, the MP Flexion Strap can be used to prevent MP joint hyperextension to facilitate rebalancing of torque forces across the MP joint to allow more efficient PIP joint extension. Acute complications may occur on device installation

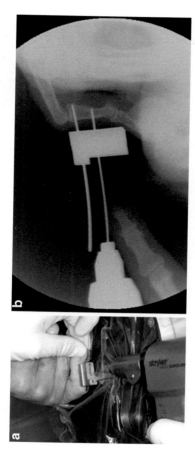

Fig. 13.4 (**a**) Proximal and distal predrill pins placement with (**b**) fluoroscopic guidance

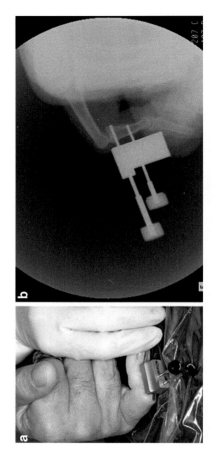

Fig. 13.5 (a) Proximal and distal predrill pins replaced with permanent screws and (b) depth confirmed with fluoroscopy

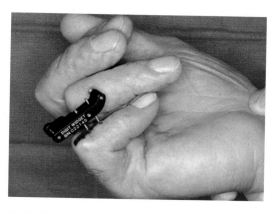

Fig. 13.6 Pin block seated 5 mm above the dorsal skin

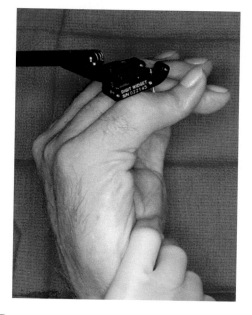

Fig. 13.7 Connector assembly and rubber band placement (Cuff and MP Flexion Strap not shown)

including damage to tendons or the neurovascular bundle upon insertion of the bone pins, tissue necrosis from excessive heat generated during placement of the bone pins, and breakage of the device components.

After 6 weeks of Digit Widget distraction, the amount of contracture correction is assessed and operative considerations are entertained depending on the amount of contracture correction and evidence of residual Dupuytren's disease [2, 10]. If significant PIP joint contracture has not been corrected and Dupuytren's disease has not been operated on previously, the Digit Widget is then removed and palmar fasciectomy is performed. If the PIP joint is straight, but significant Dupuytren's nodularity remains, the Digit Widget is removed and palmar fasciectomy is performed. Lastly, if the PIP joint is straight and supple with no residual Dupuytren's disease or excessive scarring, the Digit Widget is removed and no additional surgery is required.

The Digit Widget offers an adjunct modality for treatment of flexion contractures of the PIP joint. The ideal management of severe PIP joint contractures is still debatable, and surgical management of Dupuytren's contractures has largely been disappointing [12–14]. Literature regarding the use of the Digit Widget combined with surgery is limited [2, 3, 10]. Craft et al. showed a statistically significant average extension improvement in digits treated with distraction of 53.4° compared to 31.4° in digits treated with fasciectomy plus ligament release [2]. No studies that compare the effectiveness of the Digit Widget to dynamic extension splint orthoses exist. Other external fixation devices designed to apply continuous soft tissue distraction for correction of severe PIP joint flexion contractures have been reported. Messina et al. described the continuous extension technique for severe PIP joint flexion contractures using the "Tecnica di Estensione Continua" (TEC) apparatus where passive distraction is applied over a 2-to-4-week period [5]. The TEC device is anchored into the fifth metacarpal by two threaded pins and skeletal traction rings are anchored to the affected digits. Traction to lengthen the contracted soft tissues is accomplished by turning screws on threaded rods that are attached to the skeletal traction rings. Citron and Messina reported their experience using the TEC device as well as another skeletal external fixator device for correction of severe PIP joint flexion contractures called the Verona apparatus [7]. The Verona apparatus is anchored to the affected digit by two threaded pins placed on the phalanges on each side of the PIP joint. An Allen wrench is used to turn a gear to provide extension torque force. Both devices were used as progressive static splints before fasciectomy but the sample size was too small to make comparisons and preliminary results showed correction of contracture but overall results were worse than Messina's study. Kasabian et al. described use of a multiplanar distractor that was originally designed for mandibular distraction for correction of PIP joint contracture in one patient but the results did not show maintenance of finger extension [15]. Houshian et al. described the use of the compass hinge external fixator yielding an average extension gain of 38° at the end of a mean of 33 days for chronic flexion contractures of PIP joint caused by a variety of etiologies [16]. Siow et al. reported use of a miniature external fixator for treatment of severe flexion contractures of the distal interphalangeal joint as well as the MP and PIP joints from trauma in three patients [17]. White et al. also reported use of a miniature external fixator in 27 patients with Dupuytren's contracture of the PIP joint yielding an average PIP joint improvement of 75–37° [18]. Only one patient in their series had recurrence. Beard and Trail described the "S-Quattro" device for use post-limited fasciectomy for severe PIP joint contractures in Dupuytren's disease but observed significant recurrence (55 %) in their series [19]. Rajesh et al. also used the "S-Quattro" device for severe PIP joint flexion contractures but their method involved a preliminary palmar fasciotomy, followed by 6 weeks of distraction, and then fasciectomy [20]. Their series showed a mean correction of 22° in patients treated with PIP joint flexion contractures greater than 70°.

Currently, no long-term data exists on the role of the soft tissue distraction devices for PIP joint flexion deformities and the Digit Widget is no exception. However, preliminary data of the Digit Widget showing superior extension improvement compared to checkrein ligament release after fasciectomy, as well as no recurrence in the Digit Widget cohort, has shown promise. The current accepted use of the Digit Widget is preliminary distraction followed by fasciectomy and further studies in larger samples are needed to characterize the potential for recurrence and other complications.

References

1. McFarlane R. Patterns of the diseased fascia in the fingers in Dupuytren's contracture. Plast Reconstr Surg. 1974;54:31–44.
2. Craft R, Smith A, Coakley B, Casey III W, Rebecca A, Duncan S. Preliminary soft-tissue distraction versus checkrein ligament release after fasciectomy in the treatment of dupuytren proximal interphalangeal joint contractures. Plast Reconstr Surg. 2011;128(5):1107–13.
3. Agee J, Goss BC. The use of skeletal extension torque in reversing Dupuytren contractures of the proximal interphalangeal joint. J Hand Surg. 2012;37(7):1467–74.
4. Ball C, Nanchahal J. The use of splinting as a non-surgical treatment for Dupuytren's Disease: a pilot study. Br J Hand Ther. 2002;7:76–8.
5. Messina A, Messina J. The continuous elongation treatment by the TEC device for severe Dupuytren's contracture of the fingers. Plast Reconstr Surg. 1993;92:84–90.
6. Rives K, Gelberman R, Smith B, Carney K. Severe contractures of the proximal interphalangeal joint in Dupuytren's disease: results of a prospective trial of operative correction and dynamic extension splinting. J Hand Surg Am. 1992;17:1153–9.
7. Citron N, Messina J. The use of skeletal traction in the treatment of severe primary Dupuytren's disease. J Bone Joint Surg Br. 1998;80:126–9.
8. Larocerie-Salgado J, Davidson J. Nonoperative treatment of PIPJ flexion contractures associated with Dupuytren's disease. J Hand Surg Eur Vol. 2012;37(8):722–7.
9. Brandes G, Messina A, Reale E. The palmar fascia after treatment by the continuous extension technique for Dupuytren's contracture. J Hand Surg Br. 1994;19(4):528–33.
10. Bailey A, Van der Stappen TJJ, Sims T, Messina A. The continuous elongation technique for severe Dupuytren's disease. A biochemical mechanism. J Hand Surg Br. 1994;19(4):522–7.
11. Murphy A, Lalonde D, Eaton C, Denkler K, Hovius S, Smith A, Martin A, Biswas A, Van Nieuwenhoven C. Minimally invasive options in Dupuytren's contracture: aponeurotomy, enzymes, stretching, and fat grafting. Plast Reconstr Surg. 2014;134(5):822–9.
12. Donaldson O, Pearson D, Reynolds R, Bhatia R. The association between intraoperative correction of Dupuytren's disease and residual postoperative contracture. J Hand Surg Eur. 2010;35(3):220–3.

13. Misra A, Jain A, Ghazanfar R, Johnston T, Nanchaha I J. Predicting the outcome of surgery for the proximal interphalangeal joint in Dupuytren's disease. J Hand Surg Am. 2007;32(2):240–5.
14. Van Giffen N, Degreef I, De Smet L. Dupuytren's disease: outcome of the proximal interphalangeal joint in isolated fifth ray involvement. Acta Orthop Belg. 2006;72(6):671–7.
15. Kasabian A, McCarthy J, Karp N. Use of a multiplanar distracter for the correction of a proximal interphalangeal joint contracture. Ann Plast Surg. 1998;40(4):378–81.
16. Houshian S, Gynning B, Schrøder H. Chronic flexion contracture of proximal interphalangeal joint treated with the compass hinge external fixator. A consecutive series of 27 cases. J Hand Surg Br. 2002;27(4):356–8.
17. Siow Y, Ahmad T, Goh S. Use of a new external fixator for the correction of fixed flexion deformity of the fingers. Hand Surg. 1999;4(2):167–74.
18. White J, Kang S, Nancoo T, Floyd D, Kambhampat IS, McGrouther D. Management of severe Dupuytren's contracture of the proximal interphalangeal joint with use of a central slip facilitation device. J Hand Surg Eur Vol. 2012;37(8):728–32.
19. Beard A, Trail I. The "S" Quattro in severe Dupuytren's contracture. J Hand Surg Br. 1996;21(6):795–7966.
20. Rajesh K, Rex C, Mehdi H, Martin C, Fahmy N. Severe Dupuytren's contracture of the proximal interphalangeal joint: treatment by two-stage technique. J Hand Surg Br. 2000;25(5):442–4.

Chapter 14
The Distal Interphalangeal Joint in Dupuytren's Disease

Michael A. Tonkin and Jonathan P.A. Bellity

Case Report

Presentation

A 25-year-old right hand dominant male bartender and labourer presented with a flexion contracture of the proximal phalangeal (PIP) and distal interphalangeal (DIP) joints of the left little finger. These contractures had been evolving progressively over 7 years when he first noticed a lump on the radial aspect of the PIP joint.

The patient denied any family or personal history of Dupuytren's disease, diabetes or epilepsy. He did not recall a specific fracture, joint dislocation or soft tissue injury, but did recall a number of small traumatic incidences incurred while playing sport at school.

M.A. Tonkin, MD (✉) • J.P.A. Bellity, MD
Department of Hand Surgery & Peripheral Nerve Surgery,
Royal North Shore Hospital, University of Sydney,
St Leonards 2065, NSW, Australia
e-mail: mtonkin@med.usyd.edu.au

© Springer International Publishing Switzerland 2016
M. Rizzo (ed.), *Dupuytren's Contracture*,
DOI 10.1007/978-3-319-23841-8_14

Diagnosis/Assessment

The clinical examination revealed a radial cord on the palmar side of the left little finger, extending from the distal aspect of the proximal phalanx to the proximal aspect of the terminal phalanx. The metacarpophalangeal (MP) joint range of motion was normal. The PIP and DIP joints had flexion contractures of 50° and 60° respectively which were not correctable (Fig. 14.1). Active and passive flexion ranges of motion were normal. There was some thickening in the fascia of the first web without restriction of movement of the thumb. He was unable to place his hand flat on the table, demonstrating a positive tabletop test [1]. There was no evidence of Garrod's knuckle pads, Peyronie's or Ledderhose's disease. A presumptive diagnosis of Dupuytren's disease was considered most likely clinically.

Ultrasound and MRI scans were performed to assist in diagnosis and to more precisely designate the origins and insertions of the

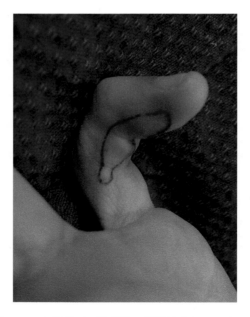

Fig. 14.1 Case report. Patient with PIP and DIP joint contractures

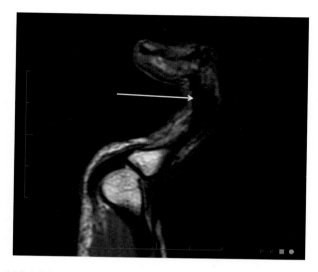

Fig. 14.2 MRI with *white arrow* pointing to the cord-like structure

pathological tissue. These found a cord-like structure extending from the level of the distal aspect of the proximal phalanx to the mid-aspect of the terminal phalanx on the radial side of the digit (Fig. 14.2).

Management

The patient described difficulty with daily activities and significant interference with function. After discussion, he chose to proceed to open excision of the palpable tissue to confirm the clinical diagnosis and to correct the contractures as best possible. Needle fasciotomy and collagenase injections were considered inappropriate as a diagnosis had not been absolutely established and the anatomical position of the tissue was likely to involve neurovascular bundles and be adherent to the flexor tendon sheath.

A hemi-Brunner incision was fashioned over the tissue along the radial side of the finger from mid-proximal phalangeal level to the pulp (Fig. 14.3). After elevation of the flaps, the cord was

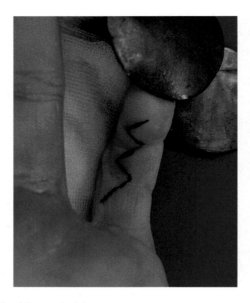

Fig. 14.3 Hemi-Bruner incision

mobilised. Macroscopically it resembled Dupuytren's tissue. It took origin from the distal third of the proximal phalanx adjacent to the distal end of the A2 pulley attachment and from the adjacent flexor tendon sheath, deep to the neurovascular bundle. The neurovascular bundle crossed from lateral to medial sides of the cord, superficial to the cord which involved retrovascular fascial fibres. At the level of the DIP joint the cord enveloped the neurovascular bundle with superficial fibres inserting into the flexor tendon sheath at and distal to the joint, and deep fibres inserting into the mid-aspect of the distal phalanx on the radial side of the flexor digitorum profundus (FDP) insertion and into adjacent skin (Fig. 14.4).

The dissection protected the neurovascular bundle and its terminal branches. Excision of the cord achieved full correction of PIP and DIP joints. The skin was closed without tension (Fig. 14.5).

The histological findings were of fibromatosis consistent with Dupuytren's disease.

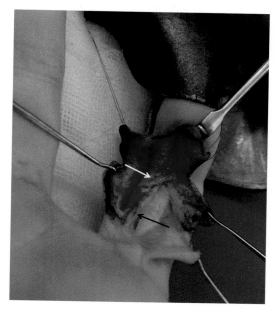

Fig. 14.4 The cord, with superficial connection to flexor tendon sheath at DIP joint level (*white arrow*) and neurovascular bundle (*black arrow*) prior to the excision of the cord

Post-operative care involved splinting and early range of motion exercises. Healing was uneventful and at 6 months post-operation there were no signs of recurrence of deformity. Active motion at the PIP joint was from 5° to full flexion; and at the DIP joint from 0° to full flexion (Fig. 14.6a, b).

Discussion

Although of a young age and without a family history of Dupuytren's contracture, the clinical findings in this patient were suggestive of the presence of an isolated Dupuytren's cord. Contracture of the DIP joint is uncommon; in fact, Ellis claimed

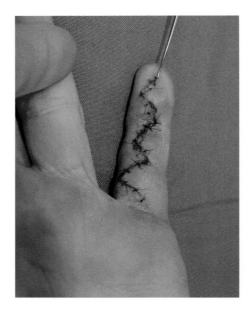

Fig. 14.5 Full correction and skin closure

that the DIP joint was not affected by Dupuytren's disease [2].
Millesi (1967) reported an incidence of 4.9 % in 287 patients with
Dupuytren's disease [3]. Anwar found a similar incidence in the
digits of 119 females [4].

A number of clinical circumstances in which the DIP joint is
involved in Dupuytren's disease have been identified. These are
as follows: an isolated primary DIP joint contracture; primary
disease involving PIP and DIP joints but with isolation to the
digit, without MP joint contracture; and a primary DIP joint contracture in association with MP and PIP joint contractures [3, 5–8].
Two other forms of involvement of the DIP joint by Dupuytren's
disease are recognised: a swan neck deformity with flexion at the
distal phalanx secondary to disease tethering the lateral band and
central slip proximal to the PIP joint, with consequent hyperextension of the PIP joint [9]; and DIP joint hyperextension
(Boutonniere or pseudo-Boutonniere). Each of these deserves
further consideration.

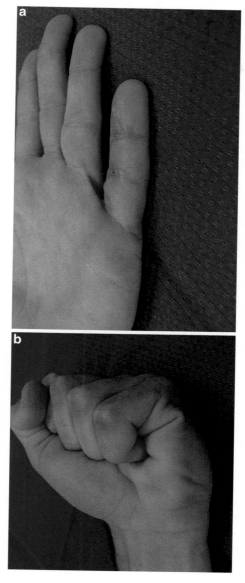

Fig. 14.6 Post-operative extension (**a**) and flexion (**b**)

Primary DIPJ Contracture

It is agreed that the most common cords creating a primary DIP joint contracture are lateral and retrovascular cords [10–16]. If the cord takes origin from the lateral or retrovascular fibres of the lateral digital sheet distal to the PIP joint, then it will result in the relatively uncommon isolated DIP joint contracture. The insertion is to terminal phalanx and skin and flexor tendon sheath deep to the neurovascular bundle but also to skin and flexor tendon sheath superficial to the neurovascular bundle depending upon whether retrovascular and/or lateral cords are involved. The contracted tissue may cause spiralling of the neurovascular bundle and may encompass the neurovascular bundle, particularly at the level of the DIP joint.

Only a small number of isolated DIP joint contractures have been reported in the literature—1 of 16 DIP joint contractures in Millesi's 1967 report, one by Bellonias and Nancarrow in 1991, one by Rao et al. in 2006, one by Zyluk in 2007, and one by Takase in 2010 [3, 5–8]. Of these five cases, four affected the little finger with the cord lying on the radial side. One affected the ring finger on its radial side.

In those digits in which the diseased cord is isolated to the digit but involves both PIP and DIP joints, the origin of the cord is proximal to the PIP joint, again most commonly involving lateral and retrovascular fascial fibres. Combined PIP and DIP joint contractures are more common than isolated DIP joint contractures. The little finger is most commonly affected—in 12 of 16 patients in Millesi's study [3]. Tubiana and Defrenne (1976) and White (1984) believed that it was the ulnar aspect of the little finger, rather than the radial aspect, which was most often affected by Dupuytren's disease, although this was not so for those cases referenced above with isolated DIP joint contractures, nor the case report of this presentation [17, 18].

A pretendinous palmar cord may connect with the lateral digital sheet proximal or distal to the PIP joint, either superficially or deep to the neurovascular bundle. In this instance, an MP joint contracture will accompany PIP and DIP joint contractures.

McGrouther and McFarlane highlighted the high recurrence of PIP joint deformities following surgery, the latter believing that this was due to incomplete excision of diseased fascia at the initial operation, although others have incriminated other factors including involvement of periarticular structures at the PIP joint and the loss of an effective extensor mechanism in long-standing PIP joint contractures [12–16]. They have stated that DIP joint contractures are more common in recurrent disease. However, there are no specific studies addressing recurrence of deformity at the DIP joint.

Swan Neck Deformity

Dorsal Dupuytren's disease presents as Garrod's knuckle pads, rarely as nodules overlying the middle phalanx, and as disease involving the transverse and oblique retinacular ligaments [19–22]. Garrod's knuckle pads are generally believed not to involve the extensor mechanism and do not produce contraction [23]. However, Addison (1984) has shown that, on occasions, Garrod's knuckle pads can involve the extensor mechanism and tether the central slip and lateral band, limiting PIP joint flexion [24]. This may lead to swan-necking.

Boyce and Tonkin (2004) have described an unusual case of a swan neck deformity in which diseased fascia coursed parallel to the oblique retinacular ligament of Landsmeer, but dorsal to it [9]. The cord inserted proximal to the PIP joint into the central slip and radial lateral band at the level of the intervening transverse retinacular ligament. Contraction of this cord caused a rigid swan neck deformity with dorsal subluxation of the lateral bands creating a secondary DIP joint flexion deformity distally. Excision of the cord allowed correction of both joint deformities.

A swan neck deformity may also be associated with a primary DIP joint contracture. The forces of the extrinsic extensor tendon mechanism, central slip and lateral bands, are concentrated on the PIP joint in an effort to extend the DIP joint, causing a secondary hyperextension of the PIP joint.

DIP Joint Hyperextension Deformity

This is the most common DIP joint deformity. A number of theories have been advanced as to the cause of hyperextension at the DIP joint and it is probable that differing mechanisms may be responsible, either occurring in conjunction or separately.

A long-standing PIP joint flexion contracture can lead to attenuation of the central slip of the extensor mechanism and palmar migration of the lateral bands with secondary DIP joint hyperextension—a true Boutonniere deformity [13–15, 25, 26] (Fig. 14.7). An extensor tenotomy over the mid-aspect of the middle phalanx may be beneficial in diminishing extensor tone to the DIP joint and increasing extensor tone to the PIP joint [13–15, 26] (Figs. 14.8 and 14.9).

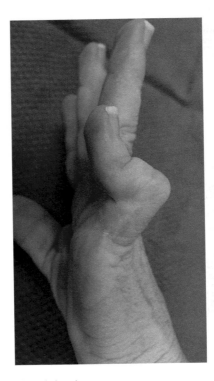

Fig. 14.7 Boutonniere deformity

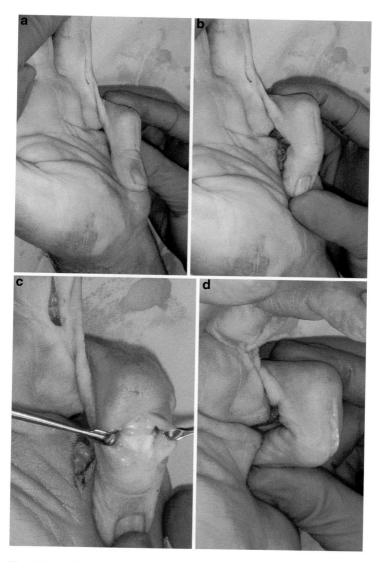

Fig. 14.8 (**a**) Pre-operative boutonniere deformity in association with a long-standing PIP joint contracture; (**b**) Limitation of passive DIP joint flexion; (**c**) Extensor tenotomy over middle phalanx; (**d**) Passive flexion increased following extensor tenotomy

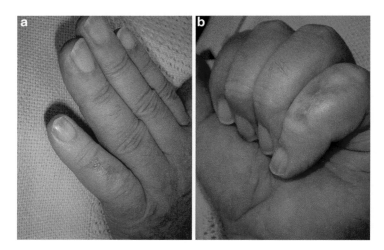

Fig. 14.9 (**a**) Post-operative extension—note that the PIP joint flexion deformity is partially corrected; (**b**) Post-operative flexion—note some restriction in active DIP joint flexion

However, even if the central slip is protected for a time, recurrence of an extension deformity at the DIP joint or at least a restriction in full flexion may eventuate.

Kuhlmann believed that contraction of the transverse retinacular ligament may draw the lateral bands palmarwards primarily rather than this being a secondary phenomenon following central slip attenuation [21]. Excision of the transverse retinacular ligament allowed correction of the deformity in his cases.

Direct involvement of the oblique retinacular ligament in the primary pathological process may create a pseudo-Boutonniere deformity with hyperextension of the DIP joint, but without primary interference with the central slip. However, McFarlane considered that the oblique retinacular ligament was rarely primarily involved in disease; rather if there was a long-standing PIP joint contracture "the fascial structures such as the oblique retinacular ligament and the extensor tendon may be foreshortened" [13–15]. In this instance, he advised division of the oblique retinacular ligament.

In addition to these mechanisms leading to DIP joint hyperextension, Hueston described a plaque of Dupuytren's tissue tethering to the extensor tendon and the middle phalanx, limiting DIP joint flexion [20].

Conclusion

The case which is presented demonstrates a primary flexion contracture of the DIP joint, in association with a contracture of the PIP joint, caused by a retrovascular cord taking origin from mid-proximal phalangeal level and inserting into the terminal phalanx, flexor tendon sheath and skin distal to the DIP joint. Excision of the diseased fascia achieved full correction. However, it is possible that recurrence is likely, given the age of the patient and the tendency for recurrence in DIP joint contractures secondary to Dupuytren's disease. The case report is used to provide a review of the differing ways in which the DIP joint may be involved in Dupuytren's disease.

References

1. Hueston JT. The table top test. Hand. 1982;14:100–3.
2. Ellis H. Baron Guillaume Dupuytren: Dupuytren's contracture. J Perioper Pract. 2013;23:119–20.
3. Millesi H. On the flexion contracture of the distal interphalangeal joint within the scope of Dupuytren's contracture. Bruns Beitr Klin Chir. 1967;214:400–5.
4. Anwar MU, Al Ghazal SK, Boome RS. Results of surgical treatment of Dupuytren's disease in women: a review of 109 consecutive patients. J Hand Surg Am. 2007;32:1423–8.
5. Bellonias EC, Nancarrow JD. Two unusual cases of distal interphalangeal joint Dupuytren's contracture. Br J Plast Surg. 1991;44:602–3.
6. Rao K, Shariff Z, Howcroft AJ. Dupuytren's contracture of the distal interphalangeal joint: a rare presentation. J Hand Surg Br. 2006;31:694–5.
7. Zyluk A. Dupuytren's contracture limited to the distal interphalangeal joint—a case report. Chir Narzadow Ruchu Ortop Pol. 2007;72:363–4.

8. Takase K. Dupuytren's contracture limited to the distal interphalangeal joint: a case report. Joint Bone Spine. 2010;77:470–1. doi:10.1016/j.jbspin.2010.02.036.
9. Boyce DE, Tonkin MA. Dorsal Dupuytren's disease causing a swan-neck deformity. J Hand Surg Br. 2004;29:636–7.
10. Gosset J. Anatomie des Aponeuroses Palmodigitales. In: Tubiana R, editor. La Maladie de Dupuytren. 2nd ed. Paris: Expansion Scientifique Francaise; 1972. p. 23.
11. Thomine JM. The development and anatomy of the digital fascia. In: Hueston JT, Tubiana R, editors. Dupuytren's disease. Edinburgh: Churchill Livingstone; 1974. p. 1–9.
12. McFarlane RM. Patterns of the diseased fascia in the fingers in Dupuytren's contracture. Displacement of the neurovascular bundle. Plast Reconstr Surg. 1974;54:31–44.
13. McFarlane RM. The anatomy of Dupuytren's disease. In: Hueston JT, Tubiana R, editors. Dupuytren's disease. 2nd ed. Edinburgh: Churchill Livingstone; 1985. p. 55–72.
14. McFarlane RM. Dupuytren's contracture. In: Green DP, editor. Operative hand surgery. New York: Churchill Livingstone; 1988. p. 553–89.
15. McFarlane RM. Dupuytren's disease. In: McCarthy JG, editor. Plastic surgery. Philadelphia: WB Saunders; 1990. p. 5053–86.
16. McGrouther DA. Dupuytren's contracture. In: Green DP, Hotchkiss RN, Pederson WC, et al., editors. Green's operative hand surgery. Philadelphia: Elsevier Churchill Livingstone; 2005. p. 159–85.
17. Tubiana R, Defrenne H. Localizations of Dupuytren's contracture in the radial part of the hand. Chirurgie. 1976;102:989–93.
18. White S. Anatomy of the palmar fascia on the ulnar border of the hand. J Hand Surg Br. 1984;9:50–6.
19. Garrod AE. Concerning pads upon the finger joints and their clinical relationships. Br Med J. 1904;2:8.
20. Hueston JT. Dorsal Dupuytren's disease. J Hand Surg Am. 1982;7:384–7.
21. Kuhlmann JN, Boabighi A, Guero S, Mimoun M, Baux S. Boutonniere deformity in Dupuytren's disease. J Hand Surg Br. 1988;13:379–82.
22. Iselin F, Cardenas-Baron L, Gouget-Audry I, Peze W. Dorsal Dupuytren's disease. Ann Chir Main. 1988;7:247–50.
23. Hueston JT. Some observations on knuckle pads. J Hand Surg Br. 1984;9:75–8.
24. Addison A. Knuckle pads causing extensor tendon tethering. J Bone Joint Surg Br. 1984;66:128–30.
25. Smith P, Breed C. Central slip attenuation in Dupuytren's contracture: a cause of persistent flexion of the proximal interphalangeal joint. J Hand Surg Am. 1994;19:840–3.
26. Crowley B, Tonkin MA. The proximal interphalangeal joint in Dupuytren's disease. Hand Clin. 1999;15:137–47.

Chapter 15

Knuckle Pads (Garrod's Nodules) of the Fingers: Painful Dorsal Nodules on the PIP Joints of the Fingers and Concomitant Recurrent Dupuytren's Contracture

Karsten Knobloch

Case Presentation

A 48-year-old male presented himself in my office with painful dorsal nodules on his fingers in association with a recurrent Dupuytren's contracture of his small finger of his right dominant hand. Prior, he underwent surgery with open selective fasciectomy 4 years ago for his right small finger due to Dupuytren's contracture. However, Dupuytren's contracture recurred within 18 months following conventional open surgery as limited fasciectomy. He had a positive family history for Dupuytren's contracture. Regarding knuckle pads in his family history, the patient was not quite sure about.

K. Knobloch, MD, PhD, FACS (✉)
SportPraxis, Heiligerstr. 3, 30159 Hannover, Germany
e-mail: professor.knobloch@sportpraxis-knobloch.de;
http://www.sportpraxis-knobloch.de

© Springer International Publishing Switzerland 2016
M. Rizzo (ed.), *Dupuytren's Contracture*,
DOI 10.1007/978-3-319-23841-8_15

Physical Examination

The patient presented himself with dorsal nodules over his proximal interphalangeal (PIP) joints on his right hand predominantly on the middle, ring, and small finger (Fig. 15.1) and on his left hand at the identical fingers (middle, ring, and small fingers, Fig. 15.2), which limit extension and were associated with pain. These nodules were palpable. Pain was provoked by palpation on the largest nodules as well as during manual exercise. In addition, he had a recurrent small finger Dupuytren's contracture following open conventional selective fasciectomy 4 years ago with a MP-joint contracture of 40° and a PIP-joint contracture of 90°, so a total contracture of 130° of his dominant right small finger.

Diagnosis/Assessment

Ultrasound examination of the nodules revealed hypoechogenic echotexture with minimal blood flow upregulation in Power Doppler ultrasound. Dupuytren's contracture showed hypoechogenic

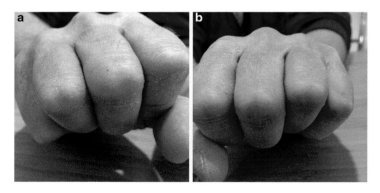

Fig. 15.1 (**a**) Knuckle pads (Garrod's nodules) of the PIP joints dominantly at the ring and small finger of the right hand. (**b**) Knuckle pads (Garrod's nodules) of the PIP joints dominantly at the middle, ring, and small finger of the left hand

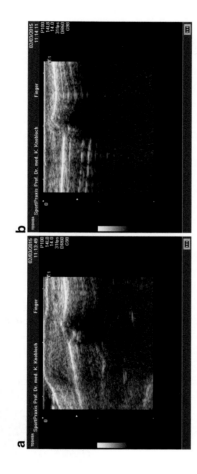

Fig. 15.2 (**a, b**) Grey-scale ultrasound for knuckle pads (Garrod's nodules) of the PIP joint as hypoechogenic mass without flow increment (**a**) in contrast to the index finger without the hypoechogenic mass

superficial texture changed superficial to the superficial flexor tendon involving the A1-pulley ligament.

Epidemiological data on the incidence of knuckle pads should be interpreted in a geographical perspective as it is the case for Dupuytren's contracture with a dominance in Northern Europe. In a northern Germany cohort of 566 Dupuytren's contracture patients, knuckle pads were evident in 6.7 % [1]. Mikkelsen from Norway reported a rate of 9 % in adults Norwegian males and 8.6 % in Norwegian females—when Dupuytren's contracture was simultaneously evident, the rate was increased fourfold [2]. In the CORD I collagenase RCT with Dupuytren's contracture of at least 20° at the MP or PIP joint, a knuckle pad rate of 5.2 % was reported [3]. In epilepsy patients from the United Kingdom, knuckle pads occurred in 42 % of epileptic males and 40 % of epileptic females [4].

Management

In 1893, Archibald Garrod, the principal reporting physician of "Garrod's nodules" from the Hospital for Sick Children at Great Ormond Street, London, UK, once stated: "*I know of no plan of treatment with is of any avail in reducing the size of the pads or in causing them to disappear.*" In an evidence-based perspective, nothing substantial has changed in 2015—there is no randomized controlled trial out yet on any treatment modality in Garrod's nodules [5].

However, given the published data derived from the most prevalent fibromatosis, Dupuytren's contracture, I proposed the combination of focused extracorporeal shockwave therapy (ESWT) as well as topical antifibrotic treatment with TGF-ß-inhibitor acetylcysteine (ACC) to overcome the pain of the Garrod's nodules [6] (Fig. 15.3). Focused ESWT was performed with a Storz Ultra device with pain-limited energy flux densities up to 0.3 mJ/mm^2 with 1000 impulses for each knuckle pad on a weekly base for three treatments. Pain was reduced from VAS 6/10 before to 1/10 after 4 weeks.

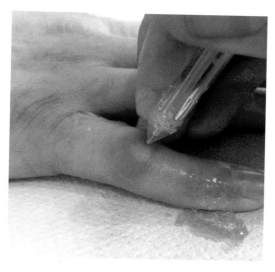

Fig. 15.3 Topical antifibrotic treatment using acetyl-cysteine instillation as a profibrogenic transforming growth factor (TGF)-ß-blocking agent limiting fibrosis and potentially reducing recurrences with a high-flow water-beam JetPeel system without pain

As far as the recurrent Dupuytren's contracture in this patient was concerned, enzymatic fasciotomy using collagenase injection was performed in combination with focused ESWT as well as topical antifibrotic ACC [7] at his small finger (Fig. 15.4). Focused ESWT has been shown to reduce pain in plantar Ledderhose's disease [8]. A randomized controlled trial on focused ESWT in nodular Dupuytren's disease Tubiana N (DupuyShock) is near to be published soon with 1-year follow-up data.

A small skin laceration at the small finger following enzymatic fasciotomy with collagenase injection healed by secondary intention supported by the focused extracorporeal shockwave therapy (ESWT). To date, the evident flexor tendon lacerations following collagenase injection therapy in the CORD 1 trial have been found at the small finger at the PIP joint level. Therefore, we suggest being aware of the complicated small finger Dupuytren's contracture when treating with collagenase injection [9].

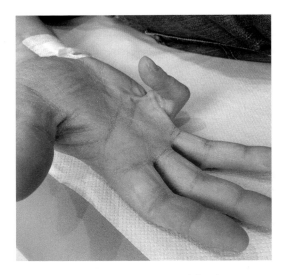

Fig. 15.4 Recurrent Dupuytren's contracture following open conventional surgery and concomitant bilateral Knuckle pads (Garrod's nodules). MP-joint contracture of 40° and PIP-joint contracture of 90° prior to combined enzymatic fasciotomy with collagenase injection and focused extracorporeal shockwave therapy (ESWT) and topical antifibrotic treatment with acetyl-cysteine

Outcome

Recurrence of both knuckle pads and Dupuytren's contracture is a potential outcome. Recurrence definition is still an issue of debate [10]. No controlled long-term recurrence data are published on knuckle pads. Given the fact that focused ESWT has been shown to reduce pain and improve function in other fibromatosis like Ledderhose's disease of the foot or Dupuytren's disease, the complete noninvasive approach focusing on pain reduction with the ESWT as well as potentially slow down the fibrosis progress using local antifibrotic ACC therapy are suitable options in terms of symptom control (Figs. 15.5 and 15.6).

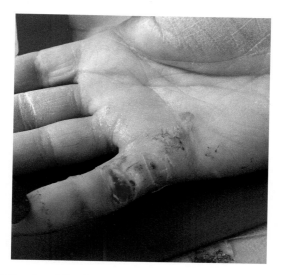

Fig. 15.5 Five days following cord breaking using enzymatic fasciotomy with collagenase injection combined with focused extracorporeal shockwave therapy (ESWT) and topical antifibrotic treatment with acetyl-cysteine in recurrent Dupuytren's contracture following open conventional surgery and concomitant bilateral Knuckle pads (Garrod's nodules)

Pearls and Pitfalls

- Knuckle pads are benign nodules on the proximal interphalangeal joints often associated with Dupuytren's contracture.
- Painful knuckle pads might warrant therapy.
- Pain and potential disease modification therapeutic options include noninvasive focused extracorporeal shockwave therapy (ESWT) as well as local antifibrotic treatment with acetyl-cysteine.
- Currently, no randomized controlled studies have been published on any treatment in knuckle pads.

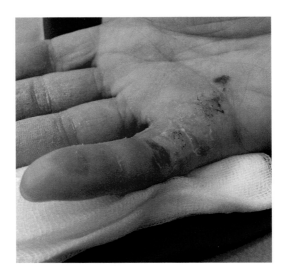

Fig. 15.6 Nine days following cord breaking using enzymatic fasciotomy with collagenase injection combined with focused extracorporeal shockwave therapy (ESWT) and topical antifibrotic treatment with acetyl-cysteine in recurrent Dupuytren's contracture following open conventional surgery and concomitant bilateral Knuckle pads (Garrod's nodules)

References

1. Brenner P, Krause-Bergmann A, Van VH. Dupuytren contracture in North Germany. Epidemiological study of 500 cases. Unfallchirurg. 2001;104(4): 303–11.
2. Mikkelsen OA. Knuckle pads in Dupuytren's disease. Hand. 1977;9(3): 301–5.
3. Hurst LC, Badalamente MA, Hentz VR, Hotchkiss RN, Kaplan FT, Meals RA, Smith TM, Rodzvilla J, CORD I. study group. Injectable collagenase clostridium histolyticum for Dupuytren's contracture. N Engl J Med. 2009;361(10):968–79.
4. Critchley EM, Vakil SD, Hayward HW, Owen VM. Dupuytren's disease in epilepsy: result of prolonged administration of anticonvulsants. J Neurol Neurosurg Psychiatry. 1976;39(5):498–503.
5. Knobloch K. Knuckle pads and therapeutic options. MMW Fortschr Med. 2012;154(19):41–2.
6. Knobloch K. From nodules to cords in Dupuytren's contracture. MMW Fortschr Med. 2012;154(19):37–8.

7. Knobloch K, Redeker J, Vogt PM. Antifibrotic medication using a combination of N-acetyl-L-cysteine (NAC) and ACE inhibitors can prevent the recurrence of Dupuytren's disease. Med Hypotheses. 2009;73(5):659–61.
8. Knobloch K, Vogt PM. High-energy focused extracorporeal shockwave therapy reduces pain in plantar fibromatosis (Ledderhose's disease). BMC Res Notes. 2012;5:542.
9. Knobloch K, Vogt PM. Beware of the small finger and/or the proximal interphalangeal joint? Skin lacerations following collagenase injection in Dupuytren's contracture. Plast Reconstr Surg. 2012;130(1):202e–4e.
10. Felici N, Marcoccio I, Giunta R, Haerle M, Leclercq C, Pajardi G, Wilbrand S, Georgescu AV, Pess G. Dupuytren contracture recurrence project. Reaching consensus on a definition of recurrence. Handchir Mikrochir Plast Chir. 2014;46(6):350–4.

Chapter 16
Arthrodesis in Treatment of Dupuytren's Contracture

Ali Izadpanah and Marco Rizzo

Case Presentation

A 69-year-old female, right-hand dominant, presented with recurrent bilateral Dupuytren's contractures requiring multiple limited fasciectomy. His last surgery involved a limited fasciectomy of small and ring finger with application of Digit-widget™ (Hand Biomechanics Lab, Sacramento, CA) device for correction of a long-standing flexion contracture (Fig. 16.1). Her preoperative radiographs demonstrated some evidence of proximal interphalangeal (PIP) joint arthritic changes; however as per patients request, an attempt to preserve the joint was elected. Following the surgical subtotal fasciectomy and application of Digit-widget™ the flexion contracture was corrected to 25°. Within 2 months, she had a rapid recurrence of flexion deformity (Fig. 16.2). Thus a decision was

A. Izadpanah, MD, FRCSC
Department of Plastic Surgery, Centre Hospitalie de
l'Universite de Montreal, 1560 Sherbrooke Street East,
Montreal, QC, Canada, H2L 4M1
e-mail: ali.izadpanah@gmail.com

M. Rizzo, MD (✉)
Deparatment of Orthopedic Surgery, Division of Hand Surgery, Mayo Clinic,
200 1st St SW, Rochester, MN 55905, USA

© Springer International Publishing Switzerland 2016
M. Rizzo (ed.), *Dupuytren's Contracture*,
DOI 10.1007/978-3-319-23841-8_16

213

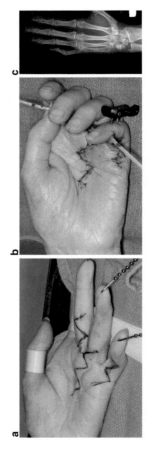

Fig. 16.1 Images demonstrating the Dupuytren's contracture and the articular changes of PIP joint prior to limited fasciectomy and application of Digit-widget™

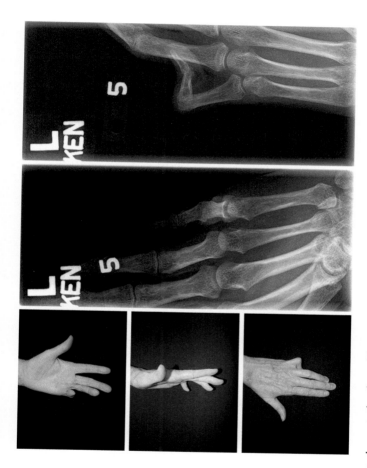

Fig. 16.2 Images demonstrating the rapid recurrence of flexion deformity after initial subtotal digital and palmar fasciectomy

made to proceed with an attempt of Xiaflex® (Auxilium, Chesterbrook, PA) injection. Minimal improvement was noted after the release and a decision to proceed with salvage procedure and PIP joint arthrodesis to address both the Boutonnière deformity and the flexion contracture recurrence.

Assessment

The patient had rapid recurrence of his flexion deformity after subtotal fasciectomy and application of Digit-widget™. Given the pre-existing arthritic changes at the PIP joint in the context of failure to correct the flexion contracture, a decision was made to proceed with PIP joint arthrodesis to both obtain a more desirable position of the joint and further prevent progression of the deformity.

Management

The initial aspects of the procedure involved a dorsal approach to the small finger. A tendon-splitting approach was then utilized; however given the extent of contracture a volar release seemed to be necessary. At this point, a small transverse incision was utilized, centered over the cord just distal to the MP flexion crease. A fasciotomy was then to allow for correction of her deformity to approximately 55–60°. Attention was turned to dorsum of the joint and using three 0.035 in. Kirschner wires, a successful arthrodesis of the PIP joint was performed.

Outcome

Patient had favorable outcome with substantial improvement in the use of her hand. At 2-year follow-up visit, she had no recurrence of her flexion contracture with good use of hand. The results were so satisfying to the patient that she had opted for a similar procedure to address her contralateral ring finger deformity with similar findings 1 year after the surgery.

Literature Review

Recurrent Dupuytren's contracture is seen in up to 71 % of patients [1,2]. Recurrence can be more often seen in individuals with Dupuytren's diathesis, originally described by Heuston as bilateral disease, strong family history, ectopic involvement, and early age of onset [2]. Occasionally it is necessary in Dupuytren's disease to modify the basic approach of limited fasciectomy, especially in the context of recurrent disease. In a study by Roush and Stern, authors investigated three different alternatives in management of recurrent Dupuytren's contracture [3]. In their results, they showed that the final total active range of motion (TAM) was not significantly different from preoperative TAM for patients undergoing fasciectomy and interphalangeal arthrodesis or dermofasciectomy and full-thickness skin graft. However patients with limited fasciectomy and local flap coverage had the best final TAM compared to preoperative values. Tonkin in a separate study demonstrated only 4 % recurrence rate after skin graft versus 42 % outside the grafting [4]. Thus, there is no consensus in the optimal management of recurrent Dupuytren's contracture. Watson and Fong in a review of salvage procedures for addressing recurrent Dupuytren's contractures discuss some of these procedures such as use of local flaps, use of skin graft, joint replacement, osteotomy, and arthrodesis [5].

Arthrodesis can provide a stable joint in a more functional position. The position of arthrodesis changes according to the involved digit and also depends on the patient's needs. As a rule of thumb, given the ability of small and ring fingers' hyperextension, the index is fused at 20°, the middle at 30°, the middle at 40°, and the small finger at 45° [4]. Thus, a multi-operated fixed PIP joint arthrodesis can provide a stable joint in a more functional position. Moberg recommends resecting the PIP joint and using a quadrangular bone peg from the proximal ulna to leave the finger in 25° of flexion [6]. The flexion at the MP joint makes the loss of PIP flexion less important. Our preferred method of arthrodesis for PIP joint is the use of multiple Kirschner wires (K-wires) or the tension band technique using two K-wire and figure-of-eight interosseous wires (Fig. 16.3). Other authors have used isolated interosseous wiring, or miniplate and screws [7–9]. Moberg also describes a dorsal wedge osteotomy for flexion contractures up to 90° of dorsal angulation.

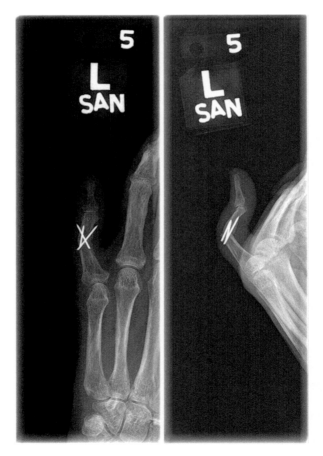

Fig. 16.3 Radiographs demonstrating PIP joint arthrodesis using Kirschner wires technique

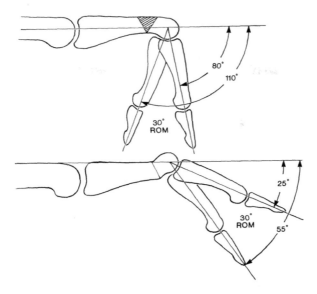

Fig. 16.4 Schematic presentation of dorsal osteotomy [6]

This technique allows the motion to be preserved in the finger with total arc of motion being transferred dorsally (Fig. 16.4) [6]. Watson and Fong describe a concave-convex arthrodesis technique in an attempt to salvage procedure of choice [5]. This technique could be reserved for when a palmar approach does not provide adequate release or will compromise the digit due to multiple previous surgeries with a flexion contracture of greater than 70° (Fig. 16.5).

Although previous studies have demonstrated absence of any correlation between Dupuytren's diathesis and recurrence rate and only the severity of preoperative condition affecting the recurrence rate, other studies indicate correlation of higher recurrence rate in the presence of at least one component of diathesis [3,10]. A lower total active range of motion (TAM) fowlloing interphalangeal arthrodesis did not affect the experienced quality of life in these patients. In general, these patients are usually well educated about their disease and thankful for merely avoiding amputation [3].

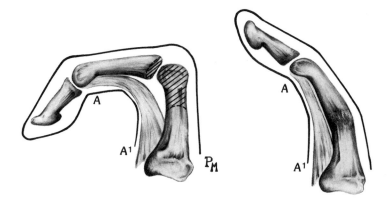

Fig. 16.5 Schematic presentation of concave-convex osteotomy to address severe long-lasting flexion deformity in chronic Dupuytren's contracture with arthritic changes at the joint [5]

Clinical Pearls/Pitfalls

- PIP joint flexion contracture release can be considered in a stepwise manner with first release of palmar skin after previous surgical interventions, recurrent cord development, joint capsule, and checkrein ligaments.
- The oblique retinacular ligament of Landsmeer may become tight after a long-lasting Dupuytren's contracture and produce flexion of the PIP joint and subsequent hyperextension of the distal interphalangeal joint. Thus, this can result into a Boutonniere deformity. Transection of the Landsmeer ligament is recommended in these cases.
- The effect of gradual external digit extensor in treatment of long-lasting PIP joint flexion contracture can be suboptimal.
- At times, the long-lasting flexion contracture of the joint can lead to loss of articular cartilage at the PIP joint, necessitating a salvage procedure such as arthrodesis.
- Arthrodesis can be an effective salvage procedure in patients in an attempt to prevent amputation.

References

1. Gordon S. Dupuytren's contracture: recurrence and extension following surgical treatment. Br J Plast Surg. 1957;9(4):286–8.
2. Hueston JT. Digital Wolfe grafts in recurrent Dupuytren's contracture. Plast Reconstr Surg Transplant Bull. 1962;29:342–4.
3. Roush TF, Stern PJ. Results following surgery for recurrent Dupuytren's disease. J Hand Surg. 2000;25(2):291–6.
4. Tonkin MA, Burke FD, Varian JP. Dupuytren's contracture: a comparative study of fasciectomy and dermofasciectomy in one hundred patients. J Hand Surg. 1984;9(2):156–62.
5. Watson HK, Fong D. Dystrophy, recurrence, and salvage procedures in Dupuytren's contracture. Hand Clin. 1991;7(4):745–55. discussion 757–8.
6. Moberg E. Three useful ways to avoid amputation in advanced Dupuytren's contracture. Orthop Clin North Am. 1973;4(4):1001–5.
7. Beyermann K, Jacobs C, Lanz U. Severe contractures of the proximal interphalangeal Joint in Dupuytren's disease: value of capsuloligamentous release. Hand Surg. 1999;4(1):57–61.
8. Rives K, et al. Severe contractures of the proximal interphalangeal joint in Dupuytren's disease: results of a prospective trial of operative correction and dynamic extension splinting. J Hand Surg. 1992;17(6):1153–9.
9. Tonkin MA, Burke FD, Varian JP. The proximal interphalangeal joint in Dupuytren's disease. J Hand Surg. 1985;10(3):358–64.
10. Vigroux JP, Valentin P. A natural history of Dupuytren's contracture treated by surgical fasciectomy: the influence of diathesis (76 hands reviewed at more than 10 years). Ann Chir Main Memb Super. 1992; 11(5):367–74.

Suggested Readings

Watson HK, Fong D. Dystrophy, recurrence, and salvage procedures in Dupuytren's contracture. Hand Clin. 1991;7(4):745–55. discussion 757–8.
Wolfe SW, Pederson WC, Hotchkiss RN, Kozin SH. Green's operative hand surgery: 2-volume set. 6th ed. Philadelphia: Churchill Livingstone; 2010.

Chapter 17
Amputation in Management of Severe Dupuytren's Contracture

Ali Izadpanah and Marco Rizzo

Case Presentation

An 82-year-old male presents with severe Dupuytren's contracture of his small finger involving his metacarpophalangeal joint (MPJ). He had a substantial flexion contracture of the MPJ up to 80° of flexion deformity (Fig. 17.1). He had intact neurovascular examination. His past medical history was significant for hypertension, obstructive sleep apnea, and multiple hand osteoarthritic joints. Functional limitation urged him to seek a medical consult with Physical Medicine and Rehabilitation and eventually a surgical consult with a hand surgeon.

A. Izadpanah, MD, FRCSC
Department of Plastic Surgery, Centre Hospitalie de l'Universite de Montreal, 1560 Sherbrooke Street East, Montreal, QC, Canada, H2L 4M1
e-mail: ali.izadpanah@gmail.com

M. Rizzo, MD (✉)
Department of Orthopedic Surgery, Division of Hand Surgery, Mayo Clinic, 200 1st St SW, Rochester, MN 55905, USA

© Springer International Publishing Switzerland 2016
M. Rizzo (ed.), *Dupuytren's Contracture*,
DOI 10.1007/978-3-319-23841-8_17

223

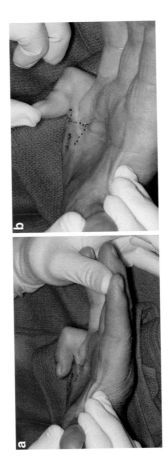

Fig. 17.1 (a, b) Images demonstrating sever flexion contracture due to severe Dupuytren's contracture mainly involving metacarpo-phalangeal joint

Assessment

A decision was made to proceed with an attempt to limited fasci-ectomy. One year after the initial fascietomy, he had a flexion contracture recurrence requiring a repeat limited fascietomy. Following his second surgery, he reformed a severe flexion contracture. Subsequently, he opted for another revisional surgery for this recalcitrant Dupuytren's contracture. Eleven months after his last surgery, he returned with similar contracture. Having failed two attempts at correction, a decision was made to proceed with arthrodesis of proximal interphalangeal joint versus possible amputation depending on the feasibility of fusion.

Management

The initial aspect of the procedure started as an attempt to manipulation of the joints under anaesthesia which was not successful. Given the extent of flexion deformity, an isolated dorsal approach for arthrodesis was not feasible; thus, a Brunner-type incision was designed volarly (Fig. 17.1). Extensive dissection was required with identification of the neurovascular bundles. Correction of the deformity to create a suitable arthrodesis proved to be too difficult. Despite extensive dissection, the skin and neurovascular structures limited correction. Therefore a decision was made to proceed with amputation at the level of metacarpal base, as discussed preoperatively with the patient (Fig. 17.2).

Outcome

Postoperatively, our patient did well with good return of hand function. He had some neuropathic phantom pain for 3 months post-procedure which improved significantly on neuromodulators and he was able to return to full activities at 4 months post-procedure. His last follow-up, 3 years after surgery, was uneventful; however, he had developed a new flexion contracture involving his ring finger.

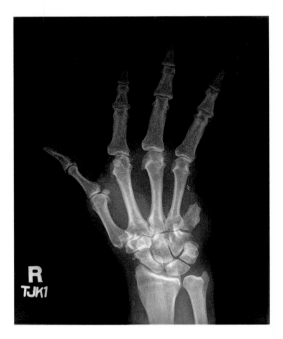

Fig. 17.2 Plain radiograph of hand post-amputation

Literature Review

Dupuytren's contracture can lead to significant recalcitrant flexion contracture and disability. Recurrence or progression of disease can occur in 2–76 % of patients [1]. Postoperative complications are also common after Dupuytren's flexion contracture release. Finger amputation for treatment of severe recurrent Dupuytren's contracture has been described in the literature [2]. The proximal interphalangeal joint, being a very unforgiving articulation, can progress to autofusion after prolonged involvement of the joint requiring amputation in some recurrent cases [3, 4]. Dupuytren's contracture being more common in the ulnar sided digits can lead to significant disability with grip and function. Small and ring fingers have been described as the most affected digits. Small finger has been also described as the most difficult finger to treat [5]. In a large series by Jensen et al., authors investigated the long-term outcome of 23 amputations in 19 patients. However, a recurrent lack of extension was seen in 9 out of 16 patients after amputations distal to metacarpophalangeal joint necessitating intervention. Painful phantom pain was seen in five out of seven amputations at or proximal to metacarpophalangeal joint. Patients undergoing amputations distal to the metacarpophalangeal joint did not demonstrate any phantom pain. Thus, the authors recommended an amputation at or proximal to metacarpophalangeal joint in patients with small finger involvement requiring amputation to decrease any chance of recurrence [5]. However, in another large series by De Semet, authors investigate the incidence of elective finger amputation [6]. Out of 31 elective amputations, 12 were indicated for Dupuytren's contracture. Eleven amputations (92 %) were performed for recurrent disease. Only one patient had an amputation at own request due to advanced age and functionally disturbing small finger deformation.

The ideal level of amputation depends on the patient's occupation and functional demands. Some studies indicate that in younger patients with more active lifestyle metacarpophalangeal disarticulation could be preferred for better grip and pinch force with a preservation of the palmar breadth [2, 7]. On the other hand, Peimer et al. demonstrated that even in functionally demanding patients, a ray amputation can lead to acceptable function with 85 % eventual return to work [8]. Thus, although a proximal amputation carries a risk of neuroma formation, a more distal amputation carries a significant risk of recurrent flexion contracture. There is no clear indication for the optimal level of amputation and a patient-specific decision should be made. Other salvage procedures such as arthrodesis (discussed in chapter 16) for severe palmar fibromatosis, recurrent contractures, and flexion deformity of over 70° should be considered and discussed with patient. In our institution, the senior author performed a total of 2 amputations out of 101 surgeries (2 %) for Dupuytren's contractures. This is similar to previous reports of elective amputation for treatment of Dupuytren's contracture [6].

Clinical Pearls/Pitfalls

- Small finger Dupuytren's contracture is more difficult to manage compared to other fingers.
- Elective amputation should be discussed in patients with severe Dupuytren's contracture, especially in patients with recurrent contracture. It is recommended to have the discussion preopartively for a possible need for amputation.
- Attempt to correction of severe flexion contracture of PIP joint in patients with recurrent Dupuytren's contracture can lead to neurovascular compromise requiring elective amputation.
- Amputation at the level of metacarpophalangeal joint or proximal to it is recommended to decrease the chance of recurrence.
- Amputations proximal to metacarpophalangeal joint are more prone to have painful neuroma or phantom pain. This can be discussed preoperatively with patients.
- Painful neuroma in these patients could be managed successfully with neuromodulators.

References

1. Dias JJ, Braybrooke J. Dupuytren's contracture: an audit of the outcomes of surgery. J Hand Surg. 2006;31(5):514–21.
2. Hogh J, Hooper G. Amputation of the little finger. Archives of orthopaedic and traumatic surgery. Arch Orthop Unfallchir. 1988;107(5):269–72.
3. Legge JW, Finlay JB, McFarlane RM. A study of Dupuytren's tissue with the scanning electron microscope. J Hand Surg. 1981;6(5):482–92.
4. Legge JW, McFarlane RM. Prediction of results of treatment of Dupuytren's disease. J Hand Surg. 1980;5(6):608–16.
5. Jensen CM, Haugegaard M, Rasmussen SW. Amputations in the treatment of Dupuytren's disease. J Hand Surg. 1993;18(6):781–2.
6. Degreef I, De Smet L. Dupuytren's disease: a predominant reason for elective finger amputation in adults. Acta Chir Belg. 2009;109(4):494–7.
7. Nuzumlali E, et al. Results of ray resection and amputation for ring avulsion injuries at the proximal interphalangeal joint. J Hand Surg. 2003;28(6):578–81.
8. Peimer CA, et al. Hand function following single ray amputation. J Hand Surg. 1999;24(6):1245–8.

Suggested Readings

Degreef I, De Smet L. Dupuytren's disease: a predominant reason for elective finger amputation in adults. Acta Chir Belg. 2009;109(4):494–7.

Wolfe SC, Pederson WC, Hotchkiss RN, Kozin SH. Green's operative hand surgery: 2-volume set. 6th ed. Philadelphia: Churchill Livingstone; 2010.

Chapter 18

Treatment of Dupuytren's Contracture in the Young

Nathan A. Monaco, Scott W. Rogers, and John D. Lubahn

History

The first patient presented at age 52 complaining of progressively worsening deformity to the small, ring, and long finger of her dominant right upper extremity. She denied any associated pain, but noted that this deformity had been getting worse since it started sometime when she was in her late 30s or early 40s. The patient was quick to point out that she remembered some of her family members had a similar condition. She also complained of difficulty retrieving objects from her pocket with the involved hand. This complaint prompted her to finally seek out care for her progressively worsening problem. The patient noted that her contralateral left hand also seemed to demonstrate similar findings. Her medical history was significant for hypertension, but she denied taking any current medications. From a social history standpoint, she did not smoke and stated she used alcohol occasionally. She denied any

N.A. Monaco, MD (✉) • S.W. Rogers, MD • J.D. Lubahn, MD
Department of Orthopaedic Surgery, UPMC-Hamot,
201 State Street, Erie, PA 16550, USA
e-mail: monacona@upmc.edu

© Springer International Publishing Switzerland 2016
M. Rizzo (ed.), *Dupuytren's Contracture*,
DOI 10.1007/978-3-319-23841-8_18

231

food or drug allergies. At the time of her presentation, she did not report any previous treatment for her complaints, aside from trying a self-directed stretching program that did not appear to help.

The second patient, a right hand dominant medical student, presented at the age of 23 with complains of inability to extend his nondominant left ring finger. He denied any associated pain, but had difficulty with fine motor tasks such as playing the piano. There was no family history of Dupuytren's. He did not have any significant medical comorbidities. The patient felt the contracture began following a minor injury 6 years prior to his presentation.

The third patient with radial-sided palmar disease and associated index finger small joint contracture presented at age 41. She reported problems in both the left and right upper extremity, but the right side was more severe. There was no prior family history of Dupuytren's or medical comorbidities. Working as a massage therapist, the patient complained initially that she was unable to place her hand flat on a tabletop. She had undergone a prior limited fasciectomy at age 33 on the ulnar two digits of her right upper extremity.

Physical Exam Findings

General examination of the first patient revealed an overall healthy appearing woman appearing as expected for her stated age. Inspection of the right upper extremity revealed contractures of the ulnar three digits. The overlying skin was intact without any break-down and palpation demonstrated a warm-well perfused distal extremity. Active and passive range of motion demonstrated a metacarpophalangeal (MCP) deformity that was passively cor-rectible to 10° short of full extension (Fig. 18.1). The right ring finger proximal interphalangeal (PIP) joint had a fixed deformity that was unable to be extended passively beyond 30° short of full extension. Semmes-Weinstein filament testing showed intact sen-sation compared to the contralateral extremity and two-point dis-crimination was intact to 5 mm. Capillary refill testing was consistent with appropriate distal digital flow. Functional testing revealed that the patient was unable to completely rest her hand flat on a tabletop.

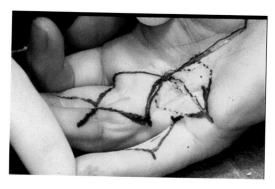

Fig. 18.1 Proposed incisions for excision and radical dermofasciectomy

Examination of the second patient demonstrated a fixed deformity about the left ring finger DIP. The patient was unable to actively or passively extend past 90° of flexion (Fig. 18.2a). A thickened cord extended from the distal phalanx proximally to the ulnar side of the left ring finger. Imaging findings were unremarkable for any osseous or soft tissue abnormality, aside from the fixed contracture posturing of the ring finger digit (Fig. 18.2b). His exam demonstrated appropriate inspection, sensation, and two-point discrimination.

The third patient had a significant contracture of the PIP joint of her index finger (Fig. 18.3). There was also partial recurrence of flexion contractures of her small and ring fingers at the time of her presentation. She was unable to place her hand flat on the exam tabletop and noted that this interfered with her ability to work as a massage therapist.

Treatment Options

Treatments options in young patients are similar to the options of older patients. At the time of the first patient's presentation, the FDA had not yet approved collagenase clostridium histolyticum (CCH) injection. Indeed, it was not until 2010 when injection of CCH for the treatment of Dupuytren's contracture in patients with a palpable cord was approved [1]. As a result, this option was not

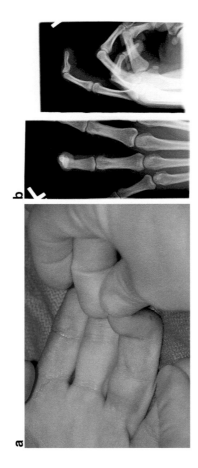

Fig. 18.2 (**a**) A 23-year-old RHD male with a fixed left long finger DIP contracture. (**b**) Associated preoperative imaging of the 23-year-old RHD male with fixed DIP long finger contracture

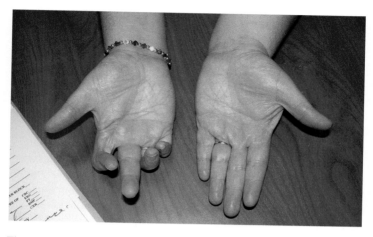

Fig. 18.3 Right sided index finger disease. There was an associated PIP index finger contracture 60° short of full extension

under treatment consideration when the first patient was evaluated. Methods that were given consideration included needle aponeurotomy, segmental aponeurectomy, fasciectomy, and dermofasciectomy. Currently, although experts may have strong opinions and advocate for one more appropriate management option in the case of a young patient with Dupuytren's disease, the evidence does not convincingly support one modality over another.

Few long-term studies report outcomes of treatment of Dupuytren's disease using needle aponeurotomy in young patients. Pess et al. retrospectively examined the results of 1013 digits at a mean follow-up of 3 years [2]. When patients 55 years and older were compared to younger patients in the series, a statistically higher joint contracture correction was achieved in older patients and a higher recurrence rate was noted in the younger patient population. The authors questioned if multiple needle aponeurotomies would improve results in young patients and the data presented in this series indicate that longer-term, comparative studies are needed to determine the efficacy of this intervention for the young patient population.

Segmental aponeurectomy perhaps has even less data with respect to postoperative follow-up in young Dupuytren's patients. Moermans' series following 175 patients managed with this technique noted an average patient age at time of treatment of 62.1 years, with a range from 29 to 81 [3]. An attempt was made to analyze the mean age in patients with disease recurrence (62.0) to the mean age in patients without recurrence (60.0), but no statistically significant difference was demonstrated. Further evaluation of the outcomes using this technique in the young patient is difficult due to the manner in which the data is reported: outcomes of the young and old patients are combined. Subsequent longer-term studies have also pooled both young and old patient outcome data [4, 5]. Despite this method of outcome reporting, Andrew and Kay suggest segmental aponeurectomy may have particular utility in the management of Dupuytren's contracture in the elderly patient [5].

Limited fasciectomy, originally pioneered by Skoog [6], has also been described in the young patient population. Coert and colleagues retrospectively reviewed 261 consecutive patients managed with limited fasciectomy [7]. From this sample, 62 patients were younger than 45 at the time of first operation. When followed over time, patients who received an operation before the age of 45 were found to undergo significantly more operations (3.8) than those who were operated on after age 45 (2.2). The average number of operations increased (5.1) if the young patient also had a familial predisposition to Dupuytren's disease. Unfortunately, other studies reporting limited fasciectomy techniques have combined data from young and old patients as well, making it difficult to draw conclusions about the utility of limited fasciectomy specifically in the young Dupuytren's patient [8, 9].

While currently the above noted interventions may be used to manage Dupuytren's disease in young patients, at the time of the first patients presentation, dermofasciectomy as advocated by Hueston was thought to prevent disease recurrence, at least beneath the graft, and felt to be the best option for treating a younger patient with widespread disease. Risks of the dermofasciectomy and skin graft are similar to other open techniques. These include infection, neurovascular injury, failure of the graft, and noticeable scaring at the donor site. Despite the risks, dermofasciectomy in the younger Dupuytren's patient with widespread disease offers an advantage over the aforementioned techniques: there is a potential for decreased disease recurrence.

Treatment Chosen

The surgical approach for dermofasciectomy in the patient with widespread disease involved marking a zig-zag incision over the most involved palmar cord. Skin markings were traced distally into the three most involved digits (Fig. 18.1). There also was an ellipse-shaped dotted line marked for skin excision along with the involved fascia. Gravity exsanguination and tourniquet insufflation to 100 mmHg above systolic pressure were utilized and are recommended for this procedure. Bipolar electrocautery was used to maintain meticulous hemostasis. Alice clamps were applied to grasp and to retract diseased skin for excision. The dissection was carried out in a proximal to distal fashion. Care was taken to avoid iatrogenic injury to the neurovascular bundle. Figure 18.5 demonstrates the depth and extent of the dissection. In addition, one can see in the image that an attempt was made to remove diseased fascial tissue deep to the neurovascular structures in order to limit possible disease extension and recurrence. Once all of the grossly involved tissue was excised, the digital range of motion was assessed. Occasionally contracture release of the PIP joint may be required to regain full finger extension. The surgeon should exercise caution to release the check rein and collateral ligaments only as release of the palmar plate may lead to joint instability and dorsal PIPJ subluxation.

In order to ensure that the digital nerves were not under excess tension, the palmar skin incisions were carried distally to the level of the volar PIP crease (Figs. 18.4 and 18.5). Near complete extension was obtained with only a slight residual PIPJ contracture in the ring finger. The tourniquet was deflated and good circulation noted in each digit. A full-thickness skin graft was then harvested from the proximal medial arm just distal to the tourniquet. The

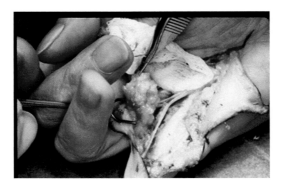

Fig. 18.4 Dissection carried down to the level of the neurovascular bundle. Care maintained to remove all fascia, even below the NV bundle, to attempt preventing disease recurrence

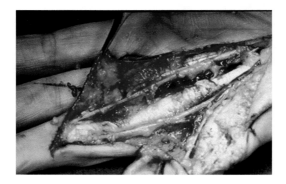

Fig. 18.5 Exposed flexor tendon sheath of ring finger. Note that the digital nerves are not under tension and the underlying tissue has been removed

graft was secured to the recipient site using a 5-0 nylon suture and the donor site closed with a running subcuticular closure of 4-0 nylon. The inner arm is a good donor site because of lack of hair and minimal scar (Fig. 18.6). A bulky soft dressing was applied at the completion of the wound closure. A final dorsal-based plaster splint was placed to the level of the fingertips to maintain the digital extension immediately postoperatively.

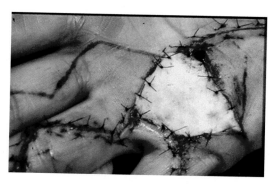

Fig. 18.6 Immediate postoperative appearance of palm after closure with full-thickness skin graft

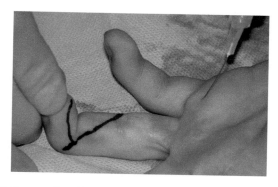

Fig. 18.7 Preoperative skin markings for an isolated small joint contracture release via limited fasciectomy. Note the local anesthetic injection site with a 25 gauge needle

   The technique of limited fasciectomy can be performed using a local anesthetic injected with a 25 gauge needle on the volar radial and ulnar aspects of the affected digit (Fig. 18.7). Preoperative markings include a utilitarian Brunner-style incision with an apex at the midaxial point of the more affected side of the interphalangeal joint. Once the tourniquet has been inflated, dissection can proceed with a 15 blade to the level of the diseased fascia (Fig. 18.8). At the level of the DIP joint, Grayson's ligament and

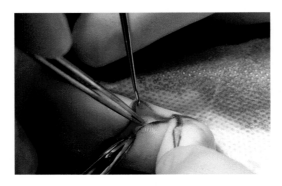

Fig. 18.8 At the level of the distal interphalangeal joint, in the case of isolated digital contracture, dissection can be carried down to the level of diseased tissue with a scalpel. Cleland's ligaments are not involved in the pathologic process at this level

the lateral digital sheet are typically involved in the pathologic process and must be excised sharply. The dissection can be carried proximal to distal or distal to proximal, as long as the digital nerves and arteries are identified and protected. Once the contractile tissue is excised, extension can typically be restored to the contracted joint. Additional soft tissue releases may be necessary to achieve full extension. Again, care must be maintained to avoid the digital nerves throughout the procedure. In order to maintain the correction postoperatively, a 2.0 mm k-wire can be placed in retrograde fashion across the DIP joint (Fig. 18.9). After adequate irrigation of the surgical site, closure of the skin is carried out using 5-0 nylon suture in simple interrupted fashion. The color and capillary refill of the digit are noted. A static, short arm splint is applied immediately postoperatively.

Percutaneous needle aponeurotomy can be done in the outpatient setting under local anesthesia. The patient with radial-sided, small joint contracture was injected with 2 % lidocaine over the sites selected for aponeurotomy. Using the technique outlined by Eaton [10], once adequate anesthesia of the digit was verified, a 25-gauge needle was inserted perpendicular to skin portal sites. Locations were selected where the skin provided a distinct

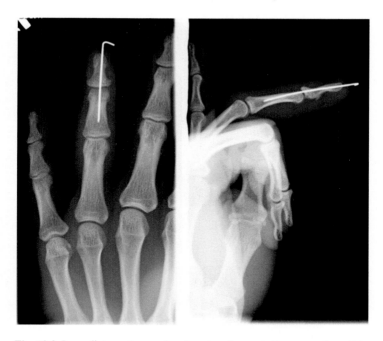

Fig. 18.9 Immediate post-procedure imaging demonstrating correction of the previously noted DIP flexion contracture

palpable cord with joint extension and were spaced at least 5 mm apart in longitudinal fashion. While more important in the palm, care was taken to avoid portal sites over flexion creases in order to limit flexor tendon irritation and skin tearing. The needle was first used transversely, to clearly define a border between the dermis and cord. Next, the needle was oriented vertically, to penetrate the cord and complete the fasciotomy deep to the skin (Fig. 18.10). The major benefit to having an awake and alert patient is that even after a block, sensation is often intact to indicate when release is occurring near a digital nerve. The surgeon can redirect the sterile needle under such circumstances. A bulky, soft dressing was placed after the procedure to maintain the joint in extension (Fig. 18.11).

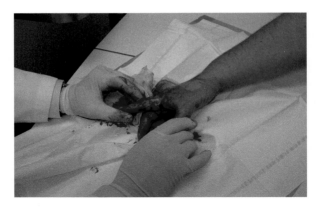

Fig. 18.10 Return of digital extension following percutaneous needle aponeurotomy

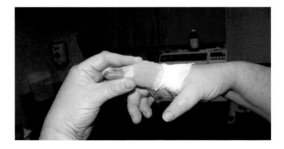

Fig. 18.11 Post-needle aponeurotomy soft dressing maintains joint extension

Clinical Course

Post-dermofasciectomy, weekly follow-up took place until the sutures were removed at approximately 2 weeks after the procedure. Once the graft had taken the patient was allowed to initiate physical therapy. The patient had good incorporation by the 3 month time point (Fig. 18.12). There continued to be marked improvements in range of motion at the 1-year postoperative time point (Fig. 18.13a, b). Over time, however, the disease was observed to extend into the small finger on the ipsilateral upper

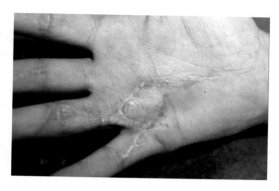

Fig. 18.12 Full-thickness skin graft (FTSG) 3 months post-procedure. Graft obtained from the forearm

extremity. Interesting to note, the area overlying the full-thickness skin graft appears disease free. Extension was noted to occur over the small finger ray. This was especially apparent when the patient returned at a 20-year follow-up for a separate complaint (Fig. 18.14a, b).

Following limited fasciectomy on the involved isolated ring finger, weekly follow-up visits took place until suture removal at 2 weeks. The static short arm splint was transitioned to an aluma-foam digital splint at the first postoperative check. Once the skin was healed, the patient began range of motion exercises in a directed hand therapy program to improve PIP motion. The extension pin was maintained for 12 weeks (Fig. 18.15a, b). The patient was instructed on twice daily pin care with 3 % hydrogen peroxide and sterile saline solution. At the 4-year follow-up, there is no evidence of recurrent disease.

Following the percutaneous needle fasciotomy, blocking exercises were recommended and improvement was maintained compared to pre-intervention status (Figs. 18.16 and 18.17). Short-term follow-up demonstrated loss of DIP flexion, consistent with FDP rupture. At 6 months, a 30-degree, fixed PIP flexion contracture remained (Fig. 18.18). Exploration, release of residual small joint contracture, and possible staged tendon reconstruction were discussed. There was some concern given her longstanding history of

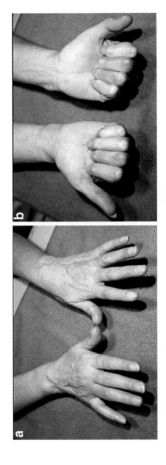

Fig. 18.13 (a) One-year follow-up, no recurrent disease to this point, almost full extension. (b) Good flexion and range of motion at the 1-year follow-up

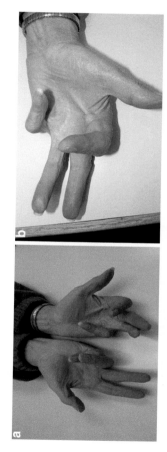

Fig. 18.14 (**a**) Same patient with 20-year follow-up. (**b**) Disease free (no recurrence) area under the skin graft, but extension noted in the small finger. This case example demonstrates the relentless, progressive nature of Dupuytren's disease, especially with onset at a young age

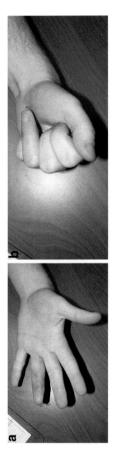

Fig. 18.15 (a) Seven weeks post limited fasciectomy and extension pinning of isolated contracture of a ring finger DIP joint. (b) Motion following limited fasciectomy and extension pinning 7 weeks post-procedure

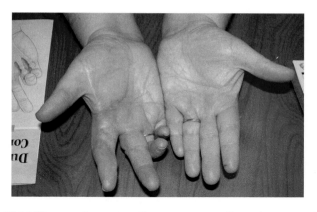

Fig. 18.16 Three weeks post-needle aponeurotomy. Exam demonstrated 30° lack of extension at the PIP joint, with active flexion to 60

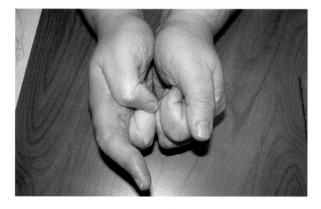

Fig. 18.17 Three weeks post-needle aponeurotomy

fibromatosis that increased scaring could result with minimal functional improvement. She was able to resume work as a massage therapist with improvement in her ability to place her hand on a flat surface, but with loss of DIPJ flexion.

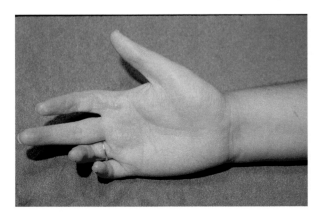

Fig. 18.18 Six months post-percutaneous needle aponeurotomy for index finger PIP contracture. Post-intervention gains noted an improvement of 30° of extension, with residual numbness and difficulty with active DIP flexion

Discussion

There is a paucity of literature regarding Dupuytren's disease (DD) in the young patients. While it is rare in the teens and twenties, the incidence has been found to increase in the following decades of life [11]. Descriptions of Dupuytren's in the pediatric population are even less common [12]. A standard definition what age defines "young" is lacking. Hueston suggested disease prior to 40 years [13, 14] and later authors have reasoned age 50 is the critical threshold for young onset [15–17]. This distinction becomes relevant considering that DD in the young may suggest Dupuytren's *diathesis*.

While onset of DD before 50 years of age is not synonymous with Dupuytren's diathesis, these terms are often related. The "label" of Dupuytren's diathesis is important for both prognosis and patient counseling. Patients with diathesis should expect a more aggressive course with the possibility for a higher chance of recurrence following surgical care [14, 18].

From an epidemiologic standpoint, incidence of early onset Dupuytren's disease is not known. Hindosha and colleagues reported on a series of 322 DD patients, 152 (47%) of which had disease onset prior to age 50 [15]. Degreef and De Smet were able to follow up with 342 patients following a procedure for Dupuytren's management between 1983 and 2006 at a single institution. In their series, they report that 48 % of patients were younger than age 50 [16]. The study noted an overall recurrence rate of 56 %, with a higher rate of recurrence in the younger population (66 % vs. 47 %). A study out of the Netherlands reported 5-year follow-up on 93 DD patients randomized to treatment with percutaneous needle fasciotomy or limited fasciectomy [17]. In this series, 33 (35 %) patients demonstrated early onset disease. When all treatment groups were considered together, age less than 50 was predictive of a higher rate of recurrence ($p < 0.005$). When considering that some of the above noted series describe study populations with almost half of the patients being less than 50 years of age, it is evident that not an insignificant portion of DD patients are younger individuals.

Various treatments of young adult patients and patients with onset of DD younger than age 50 have been described. Unfortunately, this data is often found in larger studies combined with management of more traditional/older DD patients. As such, it can be difficult to evaluate reported outcomes for thorough evidence-based decision making. Roush and Stern reviewed a series of 19 patients demonstrating recurrent DD, noting 10 patients with onset of disease prior to age 50 [14]. Among patients with early onset disease, three were managed with fasciectomy with local flap coverage, three had fasciectomy with full-thickness skin graft, and four underwent fasciectomy and interphalangeal arthrodesis. Couto-Gonzalez and colleagues reported the case of a 24-year-old female affected with aggressive bilateral disease managed with dermofasciectomy [12]. Despite several described techniques to manage DD in the young, future randomized, prospective studies are still needed to determine which technique leads to the best long-term functional outcomes.

Summary

Dupuytren's contracture, while commonly affecting Caucasian males older than 50, can also affect younger individuals. These instances are often bilateral and associated with a constellation of symptoms consistent with what is now referred to as "Dupuytren's diathesis." A number of treatment modalities exist for these complicated patients. Despite management with one of the most aggressive forms of surgical treatment for widespread disease, excision with full-thickness skin grafting, progression of the MP, and PIP flexion contractures can still occur over time. Limited fasciectomy and primary closure may be helpful in instances of isolated digital small joint contracture. The cases presented in this chapter highlight that, at present, the best available options can only remove diseased tissue. A definitive Dupuytren's disease cure has yet to be identified. Management can be especially problematic in the young patient population given the aggressive nature of the disease and high recurrence rate. Future prospective clinical trials comparing treatments such as needle aponeurotomy, collagenase injection, segmental fasciectomy, and limited fasciectomy may eventually lead to the development of treatment algorithms to treat individual patients. Such studies would need to be multicentered to have sufficient patient numbers to extract meaningful data.

References

1. Rizzo M, Stern PJ, Benhaim P, Hurst LC. Contemporary management of dupuytren contracture. Instr Course Lect. 2014;63:131–42.
2. Pess GM, Pess RM, Pess RA. Results of needle aponeurotomy for Dupuytren contracture in over 1,000 fingers. J Hand Surg Am. 2012;37:651–6.
3. Moermans JP. Segmental aponeurectomy in Dupuytren's disease. J Hand Surg Br. 1991;16:243–54.
4. Moermans JP. Long-term results after segmental aponeurectomy for Dupuytren's disease. J Hand Surg Br. 1996;21:797–800.
5. Andrew JG, Kay NR. Segmental aponeurectomy for Dupuytren's disease: a prospective study. J Hand Surg Br. 1991;16:255–7.
6. Skoog T. Dupuytren's contracture: pathogenesis and surgical treatment. Surg Clin North Am. 1967;47:433–44.
7. Coert JH, Nérin JP, Meek MF. Results of partial fasciectomy for Dupuytren disease in 261 consecutive patients. Ann Plast Surg. 2006;57:13–7.
8. Gelman S, Schlenker R, Bachoura A, Jacoby SM, Lipman J, Shin EK, Culp RW. Minimally invasive partial fasciectomy for Dupuytren's contractures. Hand. 2012;7:364–9.

9. Shin EK, Jones NF. Minimally invasive technique for release of Dupuytren's contracture: segmental fasciectomy through multiple transverse incisions. Hand. 2011;6:256–9.
10. Eaton C. Percutaneous fasciotomy for Dupuytren's contracture. J Hand Surg Am. 2011;36:910–5.
11. Mikkelsen OA. The prevalence of Dupuytren's disease in Norway. A study in a representative population sample of the municipality of Haugesund. Acta Chir Scand. 1972;138:695–700.
12. Couto-Gonzalez I, Brea-Garcia B, Taboada-Suárez A, González-Álvarez E. Aggressive Dupuytren's diathesis in a young woman. BMJ Case Rep. 2010;20:2010. doi:10.1136/bcr.12.2009.2592.
13. Hueston JT. State of the art: the management of recurrent Dupuytren's disease. Eur Med Bibliogr. 1991;1:7–16.
14. Roush TF, Stern PJ. Results following surgery for recurrent Dupuytren's disease. J Hand Surg Am. 2000;25:291–6.
15. Hindocha S, Stanley JK, Watson S, Bayat A. Dupuytren's diathesis revisited: evaluation of prognostic indicators for risk of disease recurrence. J Hand Surg Am. 2006;31:1626–34.
16. Degreef I, De Smet L. Risk factors in Dupuytren's diathesis: is recurrence after surgery predictable? Acta Orthop Belg. 2011;77:27–32.
17. van Rijssen AL, ter Linden H, Werker PM. Five-year results of a randomized clinical trial on treatment in Dupuytren's disease: percutaneous needle fasciotomy versus limited fasciectomy. Plast Reconstr Surg. 2012;129:469–77.
18. Bayat A, McGrouther DA. Management of Dupuytren's disease—clear advice for an elusive condition. Ann R Coll Surg Engl. 2006;88:3–8.

Chapter 19

Recurrent Dupuytren Contracture Treated with Fasciectomy and Skin Grafting

Reid W. Draeger and Peter J. Stern

Case Presentation

A 60-year-old left-handed man presented for ongoing evaluation of previously treated bilateral Dupuytren contracture. His right hand had undergone two prior fasciectomies for contractures of the small and ring fingers and was no longer problematic. His current complaint was his left hand. He had undergone a percutaneous needle aponeurotomy for the left long, ring, and small finger 2 years prior with nearly full correction of all of the contractures. Over the last 12 months, he complained of worsening of his contractures in the left ring and small fingers that were interfering with daily activities.

R.W. Draeger, MD (✉)
Department of Orthopaedics, School of Medicine,
University of North Carolina, Campus Box #7055,
3102 Bioinformatics Building, Chapel Hill, NC 27599-7055, USA
e-mail: reid_draeger@med.unc.edu

P.J. Stern, MD
Department of Orthopaedic Surgery, College of Medicine,
University of Cincinnati, 231 Albert Sabin Way, Cincinnati, OH 45207, USA
e-mail: pstern@handsurg.com

© Springer International Publishing Switzerland 2016
M. Rizzo (ed.), *Dupuytren's Contracture*,
DOI 10.1007/978-3-319-23841-8_19

Examination revealed stout palpable cords to the ring and small finger with associated skin puckering. The contracture had progressed considerably in both the ring and small fingers with range of motion as follows: ring finger MCP 55/90°, PIP 0/85°, DIP 0/70°; small finger MCP 75/95°, PIP 60/90°, DIP 30/65°. Two-point discrimination was 5 mm on the radial and ulnar aspects of all digits bilaterally. Garrod nodes were present over the dorsum of the PIP joints of the index, long, ring, and small fingers bilaterally. Capillary refill was less than 2 s in all digits bilaterally. Clinical images of the patient's left hand are shown in Fig. 19.1.

Diagnosis/Assessment

The diagnosis of Dupuytren contracture is often not difficult. Typical findings, as illustrated in this case, include palpable nodules and cords, usually first noted in the palm. The disease has predilection for ulnar-sided digits, but can present with cords or nodules in any digit(s) leading to contracture. Other findings illustrated in this case consistent with severe disease—Dupuytren diathesis—include ectopic lesions (Garrod knuckle pads), bilateral involvement, original onset before the age of 50, male gender, and positive family history [1]. Other sites of ectopic disease—Peyronie disease and Ledderhose disease—were absent in this patient. However, it is important to question the patient regarding these sites of potential involvement. Presence of all of the above-mentioned factors of Dupuytren diathesis increases the risk of recurrence of contracture by 71%, compared to a 23% risk of recurrence at baseline [1].

Management

In a patient with recurrent Dupuytren disease, treatment should be tailored to the patient's functional goals and the patient's willingness and fitness to undergo surgical intervention. We routinely

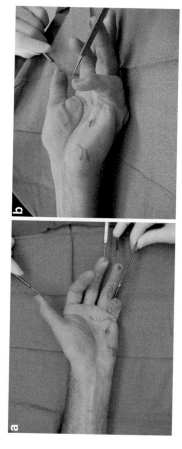

Fig. 19.1 (**a** and **b**). Preoperative view of the patient's hand (**a**: palmar view, **b**: lateral view)

involve the patient in the decision-making process for treatment of recurrent Dupuytren contracture, as many treatment options exist. These include: monitoring, fasciectomy with or without skin grafting, dermofasciectomy, surgical fasciotomy, percutaneous needle aponeurotomy, and collagenase injection.

For patients in whom recurrence is likely, surgical treatment may be favored over collagenase treatment or percutaneous needle aponeurotomy, though data regarding the effectiveness of certain treatments at preventing recurrence are limited [2]. Dermofasciectomy has a very low rate of recurrence [3]; however, it is associated with moderate morbidity as the required dissection is greater and the area of skin grafting is larger than fasciectomy and fasciectomy with skin grafting, respectively.

We selected fasciectomy with full-thickness skin grafting from the hypothenar eminence to treat this patient's recurrent left small finger Dupuytren contracture. Additionally, due to the lesser severity of the patient's ring finger contracture that was localized to the MCP joint and palpable disease without contracture of the middle finger, open fasciotomy was chosen to treat palmar disease of the ring and middle fingers. The discussion will focus on fasciectomy and skin grafting, as fasciotomy is covered in detail in another chapter.

When designing the incision for fasciectomy for recurrent disease, we prefer a straight longitudinal incision directly over the cord. This facilitates dissection down to the cord without threatening the thin skin flaps that must be raised from subcutaneous disease when a Bruner-type incision is used. Palmar and lateral views of the proposed skin incision for this patient are shown in Fig. 19.2. When using a longitudinal incision, if substantial contracture correction is anticipated, skin coverage can be difficult. Z-plasties may be necessary at the conclusion of the procedure as well as skin grafting. The patient should be informed of both of these possibilities preoperatively. Usually, sufficient full-thickness skin can be obtained from the hypothenar eminence for coverage needed following even severe Dupuytren contracture release. We favor this donor site because of its local convenience and because full-thickness hypothenar skin minimally hyperpigments.

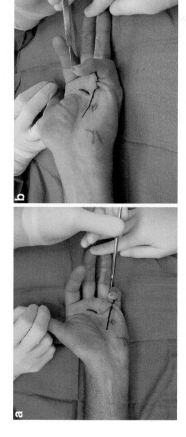

Fig. 19.2 (**a** and **b**). Planned surgical incisions (**a**: palmar view, **b**: lateral view)

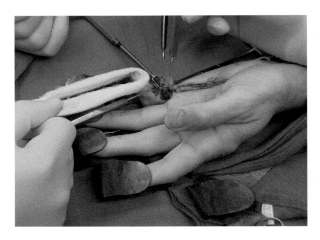

Fig. 19.3 Coloring skin with a marking pen helps to prevent buttonholing when sharply dissecting adherent cords from the overlying skin

The skin is incised and dissection is carried out sharply around the cord to free the cord from the overlying skin. Attention to placing the tissue to be dissected under tension can facilitate sharp dissection of the cord from the overlying skin with sharp scalpel. After raising skin flaps from the underlying cord, the radial and ulnar neurovascular bundles of the involved digit are identified and protected. This is best accomplished in the proximal portion of the wound in the palm. Using tenotomy scissors, the neurovascular bundles are traced in a proximal-to-distal direction. Care must be taken to dissect the bundles free from surrounding cord, remembering that the bundles may make abrupt changes in direction due to the deforming forces of the cord. When dissection is carried along the border of the digit, care must be taken not to buttonhole through the skin with sharp dissection. Coloring the overlying skin with the skin-marking pen allows the surgeon more easily detect thinning skin flaps (Fig. 19.3).

Once the cord has been circumferentially dissected, it is transected proximally in the wound and dissected sharply off of the underlying flexor tendon sheath, being careful not to violate the sheath. The cord is resected en bloc in a proximal-to-distal direction (Fig. 19.4).

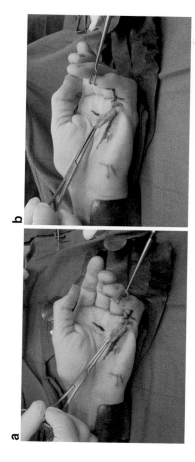

Fig. 19.4 (**a** and **b**). Cord resection in a proximal-to-distal direction (**a**: palmar view, **b**: lateral view)

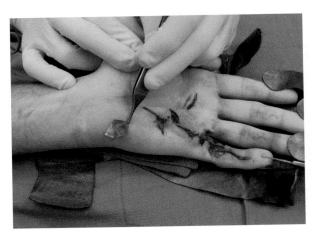

Fig. 19.5 Skin graft being sized with a cut piece of paper from a glove wrapper placed on the skin defect

Following excision of the cord, extension of the digit is possible. In cases of severe contracture, such as this case, complete coverage of the wound will likely not be possible with primary closure. Z-plasties may be designed in the palm and at any digital crease to attempt closure with local tissue.

In some cases, such as this case, a skin defect may still be present despite Z-plasties. In this case a full-thickness skin graft can be planned. We prefer harvesting the graft from the glabrous skin from the hypothenar eminence. This non-hair-bearing skin graft is similar in thickness to the resected palmar skin. It is harvested in an elliptical, football shape and can be as large as 2 cm in width and 5 cm in length with primary closure still possible. The graft can be templated with a cut piece of paper (Figs. 19.5 and 19.6). The graft is harvested in the customary fashion, being careful to defat the graft as much as possible. Defatting will optimize the chances of graft take.

The tourniquet is then deflated to ensure that brisk capillary refill returns to all digits. In severe cases, drastic correction of the contracture can lead to arterial spasm and digit ischemia. In these cases, the finger is allowed to bend and arterial inflow is encouraged with application of warm saline. Hemostasis is achieved with

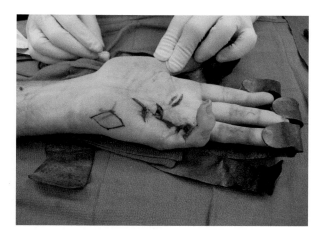

Fig. 19.6 Skin graft template placed on the hypothenar eminence to plan full-thickness skin graft harvest

bipolar electrocautery to avoid postoperative hematoma formation. The incision is closed loosely to allow egress of blood and further prevent hematoma formation. The graft is then sutured to cover the skin defect and secured with a bolster dressing (Fig. 19.7). The bolster is left in place for 1 week postoperatively to encourage graft take and decrease shearing forces at the graft site.

Outcome

The patient underwent limited open fasciotomy of his mild MCP contracture of the long and ring fingers. For his severe recurrent contracture of the small finger, he underwent fasciectomy with Z-plasty and full-thickness skin grafting from the ipsilateral hypothenar eminence. Immediately following fasciectomy and grafting, the patient's small finger passively extended to 0° at the MCP joint, 20° at the PIP joint, and 10° at the DIP joint. Joint contractures were deemed responsible for the persistent contracture of the PIP and DIP joints. Hand therapy was initiated 6 days postoperatively and the intraoperative range of motion was achieved within 3 weeks.

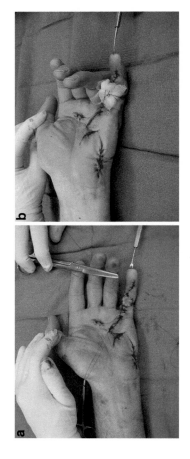

Fig. 19.7 (**a** and **b**). The closed wounds with bolster dressing (**a**: palmar view, **b**: lateral view)

Two months following surgery, the patient remained very satisfied with his range of motion, which measured: MCP 0/95, PIP 25/80, DIP 15/90. At this point he was instructed to follow-up on an as-needed basis.

Unfortunately, the patient presented 18 months later with recurrent complaints of contracture of the small finger once again with range of motion as follows: MCP 0/70, PIP 60/90, DIP 45/80. Though his MCP contracture had not recurred since surgery, his PIP and DIP contractures had recurred and worsened. He subsequently underwent successful collagenase injections and manipulations of his left small finger PIP and DIP joint contractures. He initially did well with both of these procedures, but we continue to follow him with cautious optimism.

Literature Review

Patients with Dupuytren diathesis and aggressive, recurrent disease have a high risk of recurrence following any treatment for Dupuytren contracture [1, 3, 4]. Studies on results following surgery for recurrent Dupuytren contracture are limited. One study showed that though 47 % of patients treated surgically for recurrent disease experienced functional deficits, 95 % of these patients were subjectively satisfied with the results of the revision procedure [4].

Histological studies have found myofibroblasts at the dermal/ epidermal junction of skin overlying Dupuytren tissue, which has been a strong impetus in the recommendation for dermofasciectomy for the treatment of aggressive Dupuytren contracture [5, 6]. A number of retrospective series support the use of dermofasciectomy followed by full-thickness skin grafting (either large grafts or a smaller "firebreak" graft) for Dupuytren disease in order to decrease recurrence [3, 7–9]. Rates of recurrence in these series range from 0 to 7 % with dermofasciectomy and full-thickness skin grafting.

The effectiveness of "firebreak" skin grafting in preventing recurrence of Dupuytren contracture following dermofasciectomy has also been called into question. Retrospective series have shown that dermofasciectomy with full-thickness skin grafting may not decrease recurrence rate more than other surgical treatment methods [4, 10]. Recently, a prospective trial comparing fasciectomy with Z-plasty closure to dermofasciectomy with full-thickness "firebreak" skin grafting found no significant difference between contracture recurrence between groups (overall average recurrence rate of 12.2%; 10.9% for the fasciectomy and Z-plasty group compared to 13.6% for the dermofasciectomy and skin grafting group) [11].

Another possible etiology of recurrence of Dupuytren contracture following surgical fasciectomy is the tension of the skin closed over the excision site. Two clinical studies from Citron's group support this hypothesis. In one study, patients receiving fasciectomy through a longitudinal incision with Z-plasty employed for closure had a significantly lower rate of recurrence (15%) than a group of patients treated with fasciectomy through a transverse incision with primary closure (50%) [12]. Another study found a trend (not significant) in recurrence following fasciectomy through a Bruner incision closed with Y-V plasties (18%) compared to fasciectomy through a longitudinal incision closed with Z-plasty (33%) [13].

Though agreement has yet to be reached on the most appropriate treatment method to minimize further recurrence in patients with recurrent Dupuytren contracture, surgical fasciectomy with full-thickness skin is a reliable treatment method for these patients. Open fasciectomy allows for excision of as much diseased tissue and deep dermis as is necessary for correction, while full-thickness skin grafting allows for closure of the surgical wound of the corrected digit with minimal to no tension and conveys the possible benefits of a "firebreak" graft at the excision site.

Clinical Pearls/Pitfalls

- In cases of revision fasciectomy, the neurovascular bundles need to be meticulously dissected and protected. They may be encased in both diseased tissue and scar tissue from previous surgery.
- Full-thickness skin graft from the hypothenar eminence provides glabrous, non-hair-bearing, durable, donor skin that is a

good texture and color match with for grafting to the volar surfaces of digits following Dupuytren fasciectomy.

- Dimensions of a hypothenar full-thickness skin graft should be no wider than 2 cm with a maximum length of 5 cm. Grafts of this size can usually be closed primarily without difficulty. Tension can be lessened on the closure site with undermining of the hypothenar skin to mobilize it before closure.
- For cords intimately adherent to the overlying skin, using a marking pen to "tattoo" the overlying skin can help to prevent buttonholing during sharp dissection and cord excision.
- Tension on the neurovascular bundles of the digit may compromise the neurovascular status of the digit in cases of severe contracture and full correction may not be possible.
- Despite fasciectomy and full-thickness skin grafting, in aggressive, recurrent cases of Dupuytren contracture, recurrence is possible.

References

1. Hindocha S, Stanley JK, Watson S, Bayat A. Dupuytren's diathesis revisited: Evaluation of prognostic indicators for risk of disease recurrence. J Hand Surg. 2006;31(10):1626–34.
2. Becker GW, Davis TR. The outcome of surgical treatments for primary Dupuytren's disease—a systematic review. J Hand Surg Eur Vol. 2010;35(8):623–6.
3. Roy N, Sharma D, Mirza AH, Fahmy N. Fasciectomy and conservative full thickness skin grafting in Dupuytren's contracture. The fish technique. Acta Orthop Belg. 2006;72(6):678–82.
4. Roush TF, Stern PJ. Results following surgery for recurrent Dupuytren's disease. J Hand Surg. 2000;25(2):291–6.
5. McCann BG, Logan A, Belcher H, Warn A, Warn RM. The presence of myofibroblasts in the dermis of patients with Dupuytren's contracture. A possible source for recurrence. J Hand Surg (Edinburgh, Scotland). 1993;18(5):656–61.
6. VandeBerg JS, Rudolph R, Gelberman R, Woodward MR. Ultrastructural relationship of skin to nodule and cord in Dupuytren's contracture. Plast Reconstr Surg. 1982;69(5):835–44.
7. Tonkin M, Burke F, Varian J. Dupuytren's contracture: a comparative study of fasciectomy and dermofasciectomy in one hundred patients. J Hand Surg Br Eur Vol. 1984;9(2):156–62.

8. Hall P, Fitzgerald A, Sterne G, Logan A. Skin replacement in Dupuytren's disease. J Hand Surg Br. 1997;22(2):193–7.
9. Brotherston TM, Balakrishnan C, Milner RH, Brown HG. Long term follow-up of dermofasciectomy for Dupuytren's contracture. Br J Plast Surg. 1994;47(6):440–3.
10. Norotte G, Apoil A, Travers V. A ten years follow-up of the results of surgery for Dupuytren's disease. A study of fifty-eight cases. Ann Chir Main. 1988;7(4):277–81.
11. Ullah AS, Dias JJ, Bhowal B. Does a 'firebreak' full-thickness skin graft prevent recurrence after surgery for Dupuytren's contracture?: a prospective, randomised trial. J Bone Joint Surg. 2009;91(3):374–8.
12. Citron N, Hearnden A. Skin tension in the aetiology of Dupuytren's disease; a prospective trial. J Hand Surg (Edinburgh, Scotland). 2003; 28(6):528–30.
13. Citron ND, Nunez V. Recurrence after surgery for Dupuytren's disease: a randomized trial of two skin incisions. J Hand Surg (Edinburgh, Scotland). 2005;30(6):563–6.

Suggested Readings

Becker GW, Davis TR. The outcome of surgical treatments for primary Dupuytren's disease—a systematic review. J Hand Surg Eur Vol. 2010;35(8):623–6.

Hindocha S, Stanley JK, Watson S, Bayat A. Dupuytren's diathesis revisited: evaluation of prognostic indicators for risk of disease recurrence. J Hand Surg. 2006;31(10):1626–34.

Roush TF, Stern PJ. Results following surgery for recurrent Dupuytren's disease. J Hand Surg. 2000;25(2):291–6.

Roy N, Sharma D, Mirza AH, Fahmy N. Fasciectomy and conservative full thickness skin grafting in Dupuytren's contracture. The fish technique. Acta Orthop Belg. 2006;72(6):678–82.

Tonkin M, Burke F, Varian J. Dupuytren's contracture: a comparative study of fasciectomy and dermofasciectomy in one hundred patients. J Hand Surg Br Eur Vol. 1984;9(2):156–62.

Ullah AS, Dias JJ, Bhowal B. Does a 'firebreak' full-thickness skin graft prevent recurrence after surgery for Dupuytren's contracture?: a prospective, randomised trial. J Bone Joint Surg. 2009;91(3):374–8.

ERRATUM

Dupuytren's Contracture

Marco Rizzo

© Springer International Publishing Switzerland 2016
M. Rizzo (ed.), *Dupuytren's Contracture*,
DOI 10.1007/978-3-319-23841-8

DOI 10.1007/978-3-319-23841-8_20

The original version of the book contained an error which have been corrected. The correction is given below:

Preface was not included in the original version of the book.

The updated online version of the original book can be found at http://dx.doi.org/10.1007/978-3-319-23841-8

© Springer International Publishing Switzerland 2016
M. Rizzo (ed.), *Dupuytren's Contracture*,
DOI 10.1007/978-3-319-23841-8_20

Index

© Springer International Publishing Switzerland 2016
M. Rizzo (ed.), *Dupuytren's Contracture*,
DOI 10.1007/978-3-319-23841-8

Printed in the United States
By Bookmasters